The Nature of Healing

Heal the Body, Heal the Planet

BY

ROSANNE LINDSAY N.D.,M.A.

ISBN: 0615922147
ISBN 13: 9780615922140

Lindsay Publishing

For the child in each of us,
especially my three children: Ariana, Nika, and John,
to know and use our innate gifts to heal ourselves and the planet.

Table of Contents

Acknowledgments

This book is the culmination of a healing journey that has brought many gifts in the form of generous souls who have shared their ideas, intentions, declarations, wisdom, humor, music, and love with me. I would like to hold this space to recognize and celebrate their individual power.

Much love goes to my parents whose unconditional love, strength, and support have never wavered in all the years I have been blessed to share my life with them. To my amazing doctor/healer sister, Margaret Ruocco M.D., who is my champion and confidante, who is perpetually youthful and encouraged me in the pursuit of energy healing. I am grateful for my kidlings, Ariana, Nika, and John, for the honor of guiding them while they are with me, and for their love, hugs, and spirit that feed and nourish me every day. By their example, they teach me that the children are not only the future. They are the present.

Special thanks to my long-time, multi-talented friend, critique partner, and editor, Georgia Beaverson, for her insight, support, and inspiration. Her ability to focus on the details allowed me the freedom to stream the big picture and simply let the words flow. Gratitude also goes to Martha Reilly who generously took time to review my book, and for her wealth of knowledge, her seed-planting of ideas, and her generosity of book sharing in all subjects.

My healing journey has also been a writer's journey and I am grateful to all of my gifted writing critique buddies for their years of encouragement, love, and dedication to the BIC (butt in chair) method while I raised my kids and expressed myself through children's fiction writing and poetry: Kashmira Sheth, Judy Bryan, Michael Kresss-Russick, Julie Shaull, Melinda Starkweather, the Late Bridget Zinn,

Kathleen Ernst, Gayle Rosengren, Laurie Rosengren, Amy Laundrie, Cindy Schumerth, and Nancy Sweetland.

Gratitude also goes to those artists who shared their gifts in the creation of the cover art: Photographer Paul Driftmier, Graphic artists Ariana Lindsay, Garret Wolf-Pulsiano, Daniel A. Holly (e-book), and Model Nika Lindsay, as well as those who provided exceptional comedic talent through their cartoons: artist Ken Olufs and syndicated artist Randy Glasbergen.

To heal one's self is a multi-dimensional endeavor and it has been reassuring to be surrounded by a like-minded team of health guides who came into my life when I was ready to receive them and to serve when called upon: Dr. Adam Rindfleisch, M.D.; Holistic practitioners Nicole Fenske, D.C., C.C.N., and Marcia Simler C.N.H.P.; Kundalini Yoga goddess Katie Muschelewski; Medical Intuitive Geoffrey Morrell, N.D.; Energy Workers Tina Bresnan and Mary Aldrich, among other healers. By their example of serving others with love, they showed me where my own passion lies.

To those who exemplify the hero in each of us, whom I deeply admire, and who inspire, educate, and inform with their voices, leadership, and brilliance as they stand up for truth and individual freedom and liberty:

David Gumpert, author of "Life, Liberty, and the Pursuit of Food Rights," for his friendship, journalistic skill, and vision in bringing awareness through his many projects to the plight of food rights and freedom, which has been quietly slipping under the guise of federal food safety laws;

Filmmaker and friend Kevin P. Miller, Author Jeffrey Smith, Gastroenterologist Andrew Wakefield, M.D., and Radio show host/Homeopath Dr. Robert Scott Bell, each who devote their lives in the service of others. Through their ardor and drive, they alert the public of the health dangers of chemical medications, genetically modified foods, the risks of unproven vaccines, and the power to heal, respectively. In lieu of scientific support for the safety and efficacy of many FDA-approved products, the work of these pioneers provides the tools people need to make informed choices;

And especially to my farmers Vernon and Erma Hershberger and their children, who stood up to State harassment and won their case in a juried court against the threat of criminal imprisonment for providing healing foods to private members of the farm community. Vernon is the unsung hero of our time, a simple farmer who by standing up for his beliefs, his rights, his family and his community is changing the game. He is standing up for all the farmers who are afraid to stand up. He's standing up for all of us. He symbolizes that inner strength we all possess.

Big hugs go to past companions, partners, and teachers who have nudged me along, supported me, and opened me to new ways of thinking and being even when I didn't want to hear it. Much love to those of my inner circle of influential, inspirational, talented, down-to-earth, amazing friends whose life force energy is a true gift that keeps on giving: Eva Molnar, Kathy Levenberg Ticho, Valerie Menk Raichert, Tina Kozitza Willson, Shanti Raj, Terry Carpenter, Adrianne Machina, Alex Wilson, and Michael Ellison. You are loved and cherished.

Finally, it is with a deep love and gratitude for the Earth that I write this book. Mother Earth is a teacher, healer, and champion for all life, whose soul speaks in subtle ways but is not often heard. By her example she offers wisdom, balance, cooperation, commitment, generosity, connection, freedom, healing, peace, and unconditional love. She reminds us that our individual nature is our greater Nature, which includes her peer group – the planets and stars, including the sun – whose healing rays gives us daily warmth and sustenance. Her example shows that as all of Nature lives in perfect balance, so must we.

Note to Reader

The purpose of this book is to self-empower in matters of natural health, healing, and lifestyle. Much of the information in this book is based on published scientific evidence. Other information is based on personal experience, personal interpretation, and personal beliefs. The book is divided into three main sections: Body, Mind, and Spirit, and offers writings and quotes from many authors. This is not a comprehensive book on Naturopathy. It is meant to introduce Naturopathy as the science, art, and philosophy of Nature, as well as to share related information regarding the choices that exist for everyone in natural healing. The breadth of material presented herein could be the subject of two separate books. The decision to include extensive discussion on the matters of body, mind, and spirit was made in order to offer an holistic approach to the nature of healing.

In sharing this information with you, my intention is simply to provide perspective for consideration in support or in contrast of currently held beliefs and not to convince anyone to adopt the views put forth herein. Beliefs are like ideas. They evolve as we evolve. They come and go based on multiple choices and variables. I appreciate the opportunity to share this knowledge with you. The choices presented are not all that exist and are also not intended to be specific to any condition, since each of us is unique. No claims for usage, dosage, diagnosis, prescription, or treatment are intended. Nothing herein is intended to replace standard therapies nor to be used to delay seeking standard treatment. Such decisions should be made by a client and his or her holistic health provider or health team. It is important to know that as each person is an original, there is more than one way to heal. That said, if you have a medical problem, please seek the advice of a medical doctor. And as always, do your own research.

Introduction

THE ART OF HEALING

"The art of healing comes from nature and not from the physician."

~Hippocrates

In life, art is a process of unfolding and of becoming, as unique as the artist.

Healing is an art, a work in progress, as unique as the healer. Just as art imitates life, healing imitates Nature. Nature finds perfect balance from its power to self-regulate, self-sustain, and self-heal. As a part of Nature, we have the innate capacity to heal ourselves because our nature *is* Nature.

As healers, we are here to create a life using our gifts. Our purpose is to share these gifts with others. In living our purpose, we have unlimited potential for self-expression and success. We only need appreciate our gifts, ignore the opinions of critics when they do not resonate, and listen to the Self.

There is no one-way to heal. Like art, healing is an individual experience. Each of us is unique in the way we express ourselves and in the way we see the world. We are each a canvas that brings our own imagination and unique spark. Therefore, we cannot find our most critical answers outside of ourselves. Nature, in its diversity and its resilience, is an expression of perfection that offers a glimpse of our own true selves.

The art of healing is not a competition; it is a way of life. However, to live our art takes courage because as healers we lose ourselves and find ourselves at the same time. We lose touch with our truths in the complexities of life. We conform to become part of the crowd. We disconnect from the Earth that sustains us. To find ourselves amidst the chaos, we need only listen to the heart and listen to the body. Nature teaches the most fundamental way to heal is to come into balance with our environment.

Coming into balance happens on multiple levels of existence since we are more than meets the eye. We are expressions of Nature in physical and non-physical form. Therefore, it is important to acknowledge all aspects of ourselves: body, mind, and spirit. We can begin to heal the physical-Self by eating nourishing foods from the Earth, the mental-Self by changing self-limiting beliefs, and the spiritual-Self by living in the moment.

We have the capacity to remake ourselves each moment if we choose. Sometimes we only need to step back to see our art with new eyes. Seeing anew may require refocusing our attention – looking at the big picture and looking within. We may not always like what we see. We may not want to see an unwelcome truth. The challenge is to be patient with ourselves as the vision unfolds and reveals itself. We cannot make a mistake. There are no wrong moves. There are only choices. So there is no need to rush to finish what is a lifelong creative process. It is not about getting to some future destination, since the future never arrives. It's all happening now. We are always in the present moment, the moment from which we create, discover, and heal.

Self-discovery is not easy but it is a natural part of the journey. The journey is about overcoming any doubts and fears that may arise along the way, choosing to be open to new experiences, and using our inherent gifts. An artist's journey is a healing journey.

Any journey can be a struggle in the beginning when attempting to grasp new information and ideas. Such ideas may generate conflict within. You may feel overwhelm and anger before coming to acceptance. This book may present such a challenge in the beginning. But don't give up. Simply bear down in the early chapters as you read about what happens during the body's "de-naturing process." The beauty of pushing through a challenge is that you are rewarded with a release, which comes in the following chapters, on the "renaturing process" and in the remainder of the book. You only need to bring an open mind. You'll discover additional tools in the appendices at the end of the book.

As you embark on your journey know that you are not alone. You are only unique. By your individual expression you heal on multiple levels. The key is to connect to your true nature. When that happens, you heal yourself and you heal the planet.

Chapter One

THE NATURE OF HEALING

No one else can heal you except you. Your body has the innate capacity to build, regenerate, and heal itself. Simply give it the right tools and the body knows what to do.

This fact is borne out in the way your body "reinvents" itself in every moment. Your red blood cells replenish themselves every four months. Your liver regenerates itself in six weeks, your skin in one month. The lining of your stomach renews itself every five days, your DNA every two months. Your bones build a whole new skeleton in three months, and your brain rebuilds itself in one year. Good reasons to celebrate your youth on your birthday. Your entire body rebuilds itself in less than two years. Every day is a new opportunity to build a new you.

Rebuilding the physical body at the level of the cell is accomplished on an unconscious level so that you can focus your conscious mind – your thinking brain – on the tasks of the day. According to popular science from 1980, Nobel prize winner Professor Francis Crick and his chemist assistant Leslie Orgel postulated that only three percent of your DNA is coded to make proteins to accomplish all these tasks. In their view, the majority of our DNA, the functionless, "junk DNA," with its long repetitive sequences, provided proof that the human genome is the result of a random Darwinian process rather than a purposeful design of Nature.[1]

For more than a generation this view has served to limit our full understanding of our internal workings. However, cutting edge science has since exposed the truth that our "junk DNA" is not accidental or random. It is far from the vast wasteland of non-potential that science has guided us to believe. While three percent of our DNA is equipped to fold proteins and maintain organ system function, the remaining 97 percent is our long-term memory.[2] The long sections of "junk DNA" are purposely conserved between species and do not degrade over time. They have features similar to language.[3] Some believe that twenty-two percent of this "junk DNA" becomes our memory storage of actions in this lifetime, and the remaining seventy-five percent holds our memories of our previous lives. Information from past lives comes from the memories contained within this part of our DNA. This explains why people with Alzheimer's recall long-term memories that have been transferred into long-term DNA storage while short-term memory is lost due to the destruction of connections within the brain for short-term storage.[4]

Our "junk DNA" contains the part of us that senses beyond the normal five senses of taste, smell, touch, sight, and sound. We might define these as extrasensory experiences: *telepathy* – knowing what someone thinks without direct communication; *precognition* – knowing what will happen before you get there; *clairvoyance* – seeing something without your physical eyes; *clairaudience* – hearing without your physical ears, *clairsentience* – knowing something intuitively without hard evidence; and *telekinesis* – the ability to move objects without touching them.

These epi-senses (epi meaning beyond) have gone untapped for many of us only because we didn't notice them and no one guided us to use them. So we developed a hyper-sensory atrophy of sorts. Our epi-senses are part of our *essence*, the energetic side of us that goes beyond the tiny visible light spectrum to include the entire electromagnetic spectrum. The real energy spectrum goes beyond the charted measure of 10 Megameters to 1 picometer to extend to infinity in either direction. In a sense, everything is energy. Every word and every thought has its own vibration, affecting every bone, muscle, and cell of the body. Energy healing, acupuncture, meditation, EFT tapping, affirmations, creativity, and most importantly imagination, that thing that feeds creativity, all have their foundation in this unmapped area of the brain.

The brain is ninety percent water and ten percent gray matter, a significant point when we realize that water is the source from which all life emerges. The secret of water is found in its structure, which shares the same sacred geometry with the universe. Water has memory. It is said to be the seed of consciousness. Through water we are connected to all life. The body, by weight, is sixty percent water. Around ninety six percent of body mass is made up of four basic elements common to the Earth and the entire solar system: oxygen, carbon, hydrogen, and nitrogen, much of it in the form of water. We are water, fire, air, earth, and the stuff of stars. When we respect these elements, we cannot help but tap into elemental forces of Nature, and the power of who we really are.

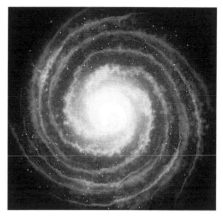

Across time and cultures, healers from around the world – including shamans, medicine men and women, and spiritual leaders – have long known that health, like truth, aligns with Nature. Nature's mystery appears in repeating patterns called fractals and in the Golden Spiral known as the Fibonacci spiral, a numbered sequence where, after two starting values, each number is the sum of the two proceeding numbers. A true Fibonacci spirals outward as the numbers continue to increase. For math enthusiasts the sequence looks like this:

$$F(n) = F(n-1) + F(n-2)$$

The sequence is reflected in the sacred geometry of an atom with its orbiting elections, a tree with its spiraling branches and leaves, a fingerprint, a pinecone, a conch shell, a tornado, the milky way galaxy, and crystals. Sacred geometry is the language of the universe. It satisfies both the left-brain's desire for logic by its structure and also the right-brain's desire for intuitive connection to the whole.

The sacred geometry seen in each crystal from the Earth reflects a unique blueprint of molecules, each stacking in unique repeating atomic patterns, each oscillating at a distinct frequency. Since crystals are able to receive, store, and transmit energy as information, they are programmable, making their possibilities limitless. The piezoelectric properties of quartz crystals to generate a precise electric charge make them ideal for computer and digital technology. However, their use for divination and protection in the ancient healing arts dates back 25,000 years. The Egyptians, Israelis, Mayans, Chinese, Native Americans, Romans, Greeks, and Tibetans all used crystals knowing that crystals store energy as thoughts, feelings, symbols, emotions, prayer, images, and intentions. This is because crystals are alive. They contain life force energy. They bring balance to a person's life. Like organs that sustain the human body, crystals and minerals sustain the life force and spiritual energy of the planet, with each crystal performing a unique function.[5] Wearing and using crystals increases life force for the human body which in turn brings more life force for the planet.

Nature in its exotic beauty, its patterns, and its miracles of creation continues to unfold beyond the level of the physical cell and into the *meta*physical, the space between and beyond the cells. As we begin to perceive this newly discovered frontier, we appreciate that true health does not begin or end in physical reality. There is also the mental and the spiritual to consider.

Understanding true health and our innate ability to heal means knowing that we possess at least two bodies, the physical and the energetic and that they are interconnected. The body is more than a chemical vehicle for the spirit. The physical body is the spirit created in bone and flesh. This means that the atoms and molecules that make up our cells each have their own consciousness. Each organ not only combines the consciousness of its individual cells but also expresses its own identity, its own intelligence. This identification is seen in the way that cells die and are reborn over and over and somehow always retain their form and their function even though your conscious self is unaware of it. The memory of the cell is retained in its rebirth.

The idea of "body memory" is not a new concept. Science has come to understand that the brain is not the mind and that memory exists not only throughout the body, but also in the structure of water, and as pure energy. Our cells are not merely physical bodies that move sodium and potassium ions across membranes to provide cellular energy. Cells are also electromagnetic forces based on their specific electric charge and magnetic nature. They have polarity and express various frequencies or wavelengths within an electromagnetic energy biofield. Consider that the movement of nutrients and fluids into cells is regulated by subatomic electric fields, of which all organ systems – brain, nervous, muscle, heart, gastrointestinal, and immune – are electrical subsystems of the bioelectric body.

Communication among subatomic systems is automatic and has been known for a long time. Max Plank, founder of quantum physics wrote, "All matter exists only by virtue of a force which brings the particle of an atom to vibration and holds this most minute solar system of the atom together. We must assume behind this force is the existence of a conscious and intelligent mind. This mind is the matrix of all matter."

Therefore, movement, behavior, and actions from our physical bodies are expressions of our electromagnetic, energetic selves. This energy exists as both potential (static) energy and kinetic (dynamic) energy, always moving back and forth between the two forms. A thought or memory can be considered static energy, whereas the movement of thoughts back and forth from the thinker – the thinking process – is dynamic. This would explain why our memories since birth are not only cataloged in the conscious brain but are alive in the deepest parts of our cells, coming back to us "out of the blue" or again and again. Thoughts inform cells. Physical form reflects soul form.

The body and soul are really one with each other. Each feeds the other for balance. As food feeds the body, the energy of that food feeds the soul. As the fertility of the land supports the physical body, the beauty and music of the landscape feeds the mind and spirit. Human nature is dependent upon a greater Nature.

If we focus solely on the physical or on the energetic, we will operate in fragments rather than in completeness. We lose connection with our full identity. True health is living at ease and in harmony with Nature and all aspects of ourselves – body, mind, and spirit – as Nature designed.

If a state of ease is by natural design, then a state of dis-ease is a reflection of our separation from Nature, an imbalance of the energy between mind, body, and spirit. Disease is not the opposite of health; it is an absence of health. Focusing on disease is limiting. Disease is a merely a symptom of a chosen lifestyle.

Likewise, health is not the absence of disease. It is the body's natural way of being. Health is wholeness on the path to self-discovery. True health reflects vitality, a clear mind, self-control, balanced emotions, creative self-expression, trusting intuition, spiritual curiosity, positive energy, and a willingness to adapt.

The point at which you find yourself today is based on your choices, habits, belief systems, and past actions. In many cases, we have aligned ourselves so rigidly with our chosen professions that we have long forgotten the person hidden underneath. In each of us there is an ongoing struggle between the ego and the authentic true Self. The ego seeks happiness in the guise of more money, power, prestige, success, beauty, or fashion. The authentic self is content with just enough. The ego feeds on prevailing opinions as gospel. The authentic self is curious. The ego is a know-it-all. The authentic self is all-knowing.

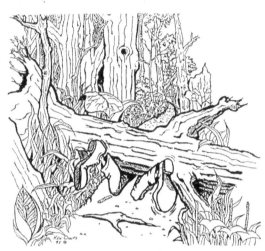

Alone in the woods…
Tom never heard it coming.

When a crisis erupts – a death of a friend or a family member, a disease diagnosis, a job loss, a divorce, a disabling accident, we can spin off our axis and lose our grounding. Depression or a nervous breakdown can set in. Since the blinders of distraction had been fixed, we did not see the crisis coming. In the chaos of change, we are afraid to question what is really happening, and afraid to awaken to the truth that has revealed itself. It is often easier to feed false impressions and maintain an image rather than to dig deep because inside we know the truth will shatter our grand illusion and take us in a direction out of our control and toward pain and suffering. After all, the ego is in this struggle to survive, not to be squandered.

But the pain does not have to define us. Pain can inform. Pain doesn't have to be a bad thing if we choose to reshape it and transform it into wisdom. The point of self-realization or "awakening" is the point at which the ego is changed. Healing becomes a choice to either continue in the same direction, the direction of the ego, or to break new ground in the direction of the soul. Choosing to purposely alter your path is done at great risk of the unknown. It is a journey into the Self from the surface to the depths, from the seen to the unseen, from the physical body to the energy of the mind and the spirit.

Fortunately, if we can move backward from full health, we can also move forward toward it. Recovery happens in reverse of the disease process. Reversal of any disease condition is possible if you focus on health. As the body is "of Nature" the body responds best to tools as close to Nature as possible. Natural health is just that. This means no chemically enhanced, irradiated, or synthetic foods or medicines that would prevent the body from aligning with Nature. It also means re-examining core assumptions we have always believed.

Seeing ourselves as a part of Nature, we see that we are true reflections of our physical surroundings. If our land, water, and air are healthy, then we are healthy. We are a microcosm of the macrocosm where everything in our outer world also exists within us. In the same way that the atom is a microcosm of the universe, the individual is a microcosm of humanity.

We also reflect the energy of our relationships. There are some people who always look for conflict. They belittle others to make themselves feel bigger. By surrounding ourselves with people or authorities who judge or control us, we feel inferior and powerless. Implicit in the word inferior is the sound "in fear." By believing we are unworthy we feed an energetic pattern of master and slave. By letting others tell us who we are we imprison ourselves. We need to ask ourselves what we gain from these relationships and why we allow them to continue. Negative patterns are built in fear. F.E.A.R. is merely an acronym for false evidence that appears real.

We need only look to ourselves for the answer. In life, we are mirrors to others as they are reflections of us. All that is needed for change is to simply see ourselves reflected in new light. Walk away from those who seek battle. The saying goes, 'the conflict they seek isn't with you but with themselves.' To find the strength to walk away, we must be ready to value ourselves and face things exactly as they are, to face up to our insecurities, and the things we've lied about to others and to ourselves. Only when we know that we are the ones we are afraid of can we reveal our unique selves and become our own masters. But we must be willing to risk a happy reflection.

Awakening is a natural process. It is also a destructive process in that we must be willing to sacrifice ego for spirit. We are not in this alone. Everyone is going through similar struggles. Everyone builds barriers to protect the overworked ego. When we discard long-held beliefs and free ourselves from fears and stories we've chosen to believe, we empower ourselves. Fear only means we are getting close to a truth. When we open to that truth, we allow the ego to rest and thereby allow ourselves to be "good enough." We relax into who we are at our core. The life force that sustains all life is revitalized and the soul wakes up and has a good stretch. When we choose to awaken, we find ourselves on the path to healing.

"We heal toward what we desire. Our desire is to be whole."[6]

~Myron, Eschowsky, shaman

The idea that the soul is an energy current of light and sound that temporarily lives in the body is known throughout all religions of the world. Over five thousands of years ago, Hindu spiritual practice spoke of this life force as *prana,* the nourishing breath of life. The Chinese call it *ch'i,* composed of two polar forces yin and yang of which all matter is composed. Islamic Sufi traditions speak of a *life force.* Jewish mystics of Kabbalah describe it as *astral light,* alchemists, light workers and healers describe an *auric field* (aura), and Tibetan mystics describe a *vital force,* the energy that connects all life.

This universal energy is the driving force behind the constellations and galaxies, and the motion behind every living cell. Aboriginal cultures and shamans today still consider the planet to be one living, breathing organism and understand that one spirit connects all things – rocks, air, trees, humans – together as equals. When we realize that matter and energy are inexorably entangled, we connect to our own greater selves and open our awareness to direct the journey of our life.

Like life itself, healing is a journey, an unfolding and a becoming, not a destination. *You* are the creator of your health and the healer of your dis-ease. Healing is a path you choose in each moment, with each decision, mentally, emotionally, physically, and spiritually.

Those who heal themselves do so on all levels simultaneously. The disease process not only begins in the cells of the body but also in the mind and in the spirit. Disease can take years and decades in the making, from the smallest decisions that we make in how we choose to express or repress ourselves, to how we choose to feed ourselves.

When we choose to eat de-natured foods, foods that have been altered from their original nature-made state so that they no longer meet the needs of the body, we de-nature the very body we live within – the temple of the soul.

When we choose a vocation over a passion, we suppress our innate gifts, the gifts that inspire us, the ones we are meant to share with others. When we always seek the approval of others, we fail to express who we are at our core. When we feel the need to reign over others we remove ourselves from forming any authentic connections. We fail to grow and thrive emotionally and spiritually.

What affects one body affects all bodies. Subtle signs appear. The "gut reaction" is our intuition telling us something is not right – it is our spiritual guidance. When we choose to ignore our spirit, over time we experience symptoms of disease in the physical body. Anger weakens the liver. Grief weakens the lungs. Worry weakens the stomach. Fear weakens the kidneys. Stress weakens the heart and brain.

Science tells us that eighty percent of disease comes from stress. Stress reflects the way in which we react to an event or a situation brought on by a stessor. Stress is merely a choice in how each of us sees, feels, and thinks about a situation. Faced with an unexpected situation, we always have a choice in how we respond. Facing the daily stressors of life, we are each the master of suggestion. Our thoughts can hurt or they can heal.

You alone embody the fulfillment of your desires or the emptiness of your negativity. What you believe and think determines your behavior and your health. In this way, thoughts become things. Real things. In the natural process of "becoming," you become what you eat, what you breathe, and what you think. You are not only a creation of Nature, you are also the creator of *your* nature. Art and artist. Creation and Creator.

"Remember, the magnitude of your life is directly proportional to the magnitude of your thoughts."

~Dodinsky

We may well believe we are in control of life until life leads us down a path we did not intend to travel. When faced with a crisis or an unwelcome diagnosis, we are suddenly forced to stop in our tracks. Every unexpected crisis presents options in how we respond. It is important not rush to judgment. We can choose to see the obstacle as a wall or as a stepping-stone. We can tune into the inner voice of self-pity or the voice of calm reassurance. Often we allow fear to consume us. We seek an authority outside ourselves: a medical doctor, a psychiatrist, a clergyman. A diagnosis is not a life-or-death sentence. It is merely an awareness. But it brings us to a fork in the road and pushes us to make a choice. How you choose to respond will set you on a new path.

Consider taking these four initial steps on the path to finding your answers:

1. Roll with the waves of emotion you experience. Any wave that pulls you down will eventually bring you back up. Flow with fear, anger, self-pity, emptiness, sadness, worry, all of them. Let them have their say. Express them. Then release them. Corrie Ten Boom, holocaust survivor and author of *The Hiding Place*, says, "The first step on the way to victory is to recognize the enemy." Once you become aware of the shadows, the pain can be surrendered so love can pour in.

2. Sit quietly and breathe deeply. Be aware that you are not a label or a case. You are a mind, body, and spirit all rolled into one, with the creative gifts to heal from within. You are merely out of balance with your natural state of being. Be what you are. Accept that you are everything you need. As psychotherapist, Nathaniel Branden writes, "The first step is awareness. The second step is acceptance."

3. Refuse to be a captive of your environment. See the situation as a ball of energy from which you can detach as easily as you would cut a cord. Cutting energetic cords allows you to defuse the situation so you can think clearly. Take a few more deep breaths, then,

4. See your new awareness as a wake-up call to make some lifestyle changes. Any imbalance is a sign that asks us to shift perspective. This is a time to crystallize who you are apart from your life. In the performance of your life, the spotlight shines

on you. Feeling lost or empty has its benefits. Long-suppressed passions and dreams may push their way to the surface to find new life – they now have the space to do so. Do not bury them again. Act on them.

"Life does not always give you what you want, but if you look closely you will see that it gives you what you need for growth."

~Leon Brown

That moment of awareness does many positive things. It allows you to move out of your head and into your heart. It forces you to slow down to be present in the moment. In this moment you discover what is important. Material possessions – the car, the house, the clothes, the jewelry, the job, the partner – are not on the list. They cannot fill the void. They never could. There is only one thing that can. That thing is found within you. It is your own essence, your spirit, the Source from which all things come. Some call this essence God, Creator, Allah, Great Mystery Nature, Oneness, Collective Consciousness, Universe, All That Is, or simply Source.

The Source of who we are is found by living in the moment. The moment is found in silence. Silence is found when we go within ourselves through prayer and meditation and we are brought to the still space between our thoughts, to our center. In meditation, we focus on the breath. In breathing in and out we alter our conscious awareness and relax. In this calm, focused state we are fully present. This place of inner peace grounds us and quiets body, mind, and spirit, simultaneously. We slow down long enough to rediscover buried treasures, perhaps hidden by the child we left behind years ago on our quest to grow up. We align with our higher spiritual self, our divine nature. We create the space to relax in the silence to receive answers.

In this space of quietude, it is important to release all expectations and judgments and be open to the experience. As we forfeit judgments of fear, anger, guilt, apathy, greed, jealousy, and pride we open to joy, wisdom, creativity, self-worth, and love. They have all been here waiting for us. With practice, we are able to mourn any loss or lack we feel and release it. We separate what is real from what is unreal. We discover that no one else has the power to make us happy. We create it for ourselves. In the process, we draw those caregivers to us who are like-minded and have our best interests at heart. We are not so independent that we cannot lean on others for support. After all, we are all here for each other.

It is important not to tell yourself that you are "living with dis-ease" because at some level that notion is a self-fulfilling prophecy. By focusing on dis-ease, you fail to find true health. By changing belief systems, health and wellness become possible. Until we learn to stop the chatter in our heads, we will forever be talked into fear.

Meditation provides a path to quiet the ego. When the ego is comforted, fear has nowhere to live. Meditation can take many forms: your favorite music, guided meditation (CD), a walk in Nature, yoga, dancing, knitting, drawing, or writing. If you want to reduce the impact of recurring anxiety, you might consider meditation as a regular practice. The ability to quiet the mind varies with each of us so it is important to be gentle with yourself no matter what the experience. Make time to sit quietly, close your eyes, and become aware of the sensations of your body. Focus on your breath and allow all thoughts, aches, emotions, and sounds to come and go like waves. Whatever they are simply be aware of them and let them be. Always return your focus to the breath and remember that it is "meditation practice" not "meditation perfect."

You can also try writing new goals down on paper and journal your feelings. Write letters to people in your life expressing how you feel. No need to send them, just get your feelings down and out. The act of writing down feelings and thoughts transfers emotions trapped in the body to lighten the load.

Listen to your heart and to what feels right. Embody the fulfillment of your dreams to be whole. Value your true worth. Your mission should you choose to accept it, is to see this crisis or diagnosis as a gift to heal.

Chapter Two

THE DE-NATURING PROCESS

When we disconnect from Nature we suffer from Nature deficiency. Author Richard Louv, in his book *Last Child in the Woods* first coined the term "Nature deficit disorder" to describe a condition we as a society have developed as a result of being detached from our natural environment. Over a few generations, we have eschewed family farming for industrial farming, traded gardening for computer gaming, and given up cooking for cooking shows. To satisfy our appetite for "convenience foods" we have become ignorant of the origin of real food. We have neglected the soil and lost the seeds of health it once offered.

In the process, we have become a nation of chronic disease statistics where our children are the latest casualties. When we fail to nurture our environment, we fail to sustain ourselves. We search for a cure so we can get on with the business of living never stopping to consider that living is not a business and the power to heal is not found outside of Self.

Today, most people are more than willing to give up their power to the educated guess of others. We trust the opinions of people with degrees who do not know us personally. After all, they are paid to give us answers since we couldn't possibly be an authority on what ails us. Perhaps we have been conditioned to fear our own intuition and distrust our ability to find our own answers.

Instead we seek answers from a system that represents averages of groups; more specifically, averages of groups of ill people. This system of averages fails at the outset to help us find balance because each of us has a unique physiology. We are each a true original with our own gene pool, living in our own fish bowl, with our own sensibilities. As such, no two people will exhibit the same combination of symptoms. The question we should be asking is if we are all indeed individuals, why should we allow a system to treat as if we are all the same?

The hierarchical system of health care is "disease-based," constrained by regulatory policies and paperwork that have compromised communication and trust between doctor and patient. If your tests do not fall within prescribed ranges you are labeled "idiopathic," meaning "we don't know." There is no inquiry into causal factors and there is no recommendation for follow-up even if you are experiencing symptoms. There is little or no discussion on prevention.

If you do become a "case," you are given a number, uploaded into the system, and mapped into a grid that separates body and mind into compartments and subspecialties. The system provides individual experts who manage your organ systems as if each organ functions in a void onto itself. You are prescribed a drug that comes with a long list of known negative side effects, of which you are not informed unless you read the package insert or watch TV commercials sponsored by the pharmaceutical industry.

The TV commercials encourage you to ask your doctor if the advertised medication is right for you. You go to the doctor expecting you will not leave empty-handed. What you do not know is that the drug contains inorganic compounds the body cannot easily process. The compounds interrupt the body's equilibrium and cause nutrient deficiencies that are not disclosed to you. You are not told if you will ever be able to come off of the medication that is not designed to cure you. Before long, there is a collection of pill bottles taking up space in the medicine cabinet.

The system labels us and controls our symptoms temporarily at the cost of maintaining dis-ease. We have been convinced to take a pill for a little relief so we can continue on with our lives as if nothing happened. No need to make any drastic changes. After all, we are not alone; we belong to the "herd." The latest peer-reviewed study "proves" the average person is sick and takes more than one medication.

If the expert diagnosis is meant to heal then why do patients continue taking medications for the rest of their lives? Why don't the experts explain why the pain in the lower back never leaves or why it has moved to the shoulder? If there is a "standard of care" in medicine, should we believe a second opinion even if it contradicts the first? Are we to believe that the benefits outweigh the risks when the insert has a black box warning showing a skull and crossbones? If our symptoms do not fall within flagged ranges and they tell us it's all in our minds, do we take their anti-depressants?

Maybe it *is* all in our minds.

The Tarahumara Indians in the Sierra Madre mountains of Mexico believe a person's own inner belief is the vital factor in the healing process, regardless of the ritual employed by the therapist healer. Two essential factors in the doctor-patient relationship are the patient's belief in the healer, and the healer's belief in the ritual. "Common ground, shared by both patient and healer is their faith in the existence of a universal power, which can induce an ailing body to heal," describes Dr. Irving Oyle, author of *The Healing Mind*. Oyle says, "The fallacy of technology dictates we can fix people, repair the body as we would a machine, when the simple fact is that the body has the ability to heal itself."

The western view to preserve life at any cost may be viewed as re-sisting death by some cultures since a doctor's idea about what is right is not necessarily the same as what is in the patient's best interest. Fighting death with technology is not only cost prohibitive but may end up working against the greater good.

Ironically, western allopathic medicine well understands the power of the mind when it comes to healing. Medicine's sole focus on patent-ed drug therapies is based on the mind-body medicine of the Placebo Effect, the mind convincing the body the drug will work. Science cred-its up to seventy-five percent of a pill's effectiveness to the belief of the patient that the drug will heal the body.[7] A recent case-control study further showed a dose-dependent response for a placebo in which the more attention patients received, even if all treatments were faked, the better they tended to fare. This provided hard evidence and legitima-cy to the placebo effect, showing that rituals and drugs use the same biochemical pathways to influence a patient's brain to heal the body.[8]

Just as the placebo effect can influence our reaction to a drug's effectiveness, the nocebo effect, shows the opposite – how an expecta-tion of side effects can cause us to experience those as well. Imagine being told that in taking a drug for an enlarged prostate you might also experience the side effect of erectile dysfunction. The "not so hard" evidence was experienced by forty percent of the group that was told of this effect, versus only fifteen percent of the group not told.[9]

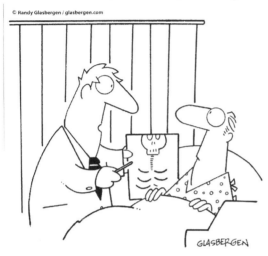

"Your X-ray showed a broken rib, but we fixed it with Photoshop."

There is no medical definition of the term "standard of care" so often used in medical literature, although the term is established in law, defined as "the caution that a reasonable person in similar circumstances would exercise in providing care to a patient.[10] Currently, it is unknown how many patients truly benefit from long-term standard medical intervention. According to the *Journal of the American Medical Association* (*JAMA*), the number of medical-induced deaths totals in the hundreds of thousands annually from approved prescription drugs, infections from drug-resistant bacteria, hospital infections, unnecessary surgeries, doctor errors, and chemotherapy.[11]

A sobering analysis of studies published in the prestigious *New England Journal of Medicine* found that forty percent (146 practices) of current medical procedures – screening tests, diagnostic tests, medication, and surgery – showed no benefit. Findings were reversed, meaning they never worked in the first place based on faulty data.[12] "Not only are millions of screen-detected abnormalities not 'cancer' in the first place but even those which can be considered fast-growing are often being driven into greater malignancy by the conventional chemotherapy, radiation and surgery-based standard of cancer care itself."[13] If anything can be gained from this revelation perhaps it is that when it comes to trusting the next cancer breakthrough, less is more.

Collateral damage of the system also affects those who unknowingly expose themselves to forced medication through fluoridation of the public water supply. In addition to drinking toxic halides of fluoride and chlorine (and bromine from pesticide runoff), people ingest prescription drugs – hormones and anti-depressants – that are flushed down toilets and recharged to watersheds. Drug residues and heavy metals from contaminated water are carried in run-off from homes and industry into plants and herbs, eventually making their way into meat and dairy products.

The efficacy of any healing system must be measured and directly proportional to the total well-being and health of the patient *and* the planet, one that will not cause harm or make things worse. Perhaps the medical Hippocratic Oath to "First, do no harm" should be reviewed and replaced by the Precautionary Principle – one version of which states: "When an activity raises the threats of harm to human health or the environment, precautionary measures should be taken even if some cause and effect relationships are not fully established scientifically."[14]

There is a social responsibility to protect all life from exposure to harm, but for too long we have swallowed the advice of experts and allowed scientific consensus to act as both judge and jury to decide for us. Government drug approval is based on studies funded by the very pharmaceutical companies that sell their own products, a clear conflict of interest.

The global pharmaceutical industry is not completely immune from the consequences of criminal wrongdoing.[15] While several high-profile scandals have undermined public trust, the fines imposed are only a slap on the wrist to a monopoly industry where no person takes responsibility, no one is penalized, and money flows back to government which continues to approve new drugs from the same companies. Nothing changes in a system where fraud is so rewarding.[16]

Over one hundred years ago, the American Medical Association (AMA) ushered in the growth of the Medical Industrial Complex along with the simultaneous suppression of herbal and natural medicine. The transition to pharmaceuticals locked in the germ as the basis for all sickness and encouraged us to sterilize all surfaces and remain indoors. Through language and repetition, medicine turns the body into the enemy that mounts an attack against us. The monopoly of drug-based medicine teaches us to demand the quick-fix drug or vaccine instead of encouraging the body to rest and heal in its own time. Doctors warn us against the healing rays of the sun, an important source of vitamin D3 (a natural steroid hormone), in favor of chemical-based sunscreens. In the span of one century, fear-based science has separated us from our roots.

In losing our connection to Nature, we have grown dependent on those who have patented Nature. The system promotes artificial enhancement over personal responsibility. We are made to believe that things will get better without our participation. Jonathan Emord is the only constitutional attorney who has taken on the Food and Drug Agency eight times in court and won eight times. In his book *Global Censorship of Health Information*, Emord conveys that we have lost the right to receive information and make decisions for our life. We've lost a competitive marketplace that allows for choice. We've lost our sovereignty.[17]

Many nations suffer from rising violence, crime, addiction, divorce, and health costs all fueled by epidemic levels of chronic stress that we attempt to suppress and ignore in the name of scientific breakthroughs. Rising disease rates and health costs alone should make us question whether the system is working in our favor. At the very least it should make us question what options are available to take us in a new direction.

If there is one thing we can change, it is our belief system. We can choose not to believe claims by authority figures and institutions telling us they are here to protect us. We can choose to accept that Earth's resources; the plants, water, air, and energy are all here for us to share in, and not a commodity to be owned by a few and sold for a profit.

What the system doesn't want us to know is that we are each an authority. We are each our own best protectors. We are all in this together. What is good for the few is good for us all. Fear is the only enemy. If there are injustices and imbalances in our environment, then we allow them to continue when we do nothing to change them, out of fear. We allow fear to control our beliefs and our behaviors. Instead, fear can inform us. It can cause us to think differently and take us in a new direction. We are our own best supporters and our own worst enemies. Therefore, in matters of health or wealth, the only ones standing in the way of success is us. With nothing to fear there is nothing to lose.

Our power to heal is greater than we have been led to believe. Each of us is born with everything we need. How healthy we are depends on how we choose to live our lives on a daily basis. All we have to do is put down the purple pill and step away from the medicine cabinet. Truth is always simple. We only need to connect to our inner Self, stand in our power, and trust that we know what is best for us.

Healing the physical Self is one step that helps bring all aspects of ourselves into alignment. We do this generally through: 1) detoxification of our blood, cells, and organ systems and, 2) nutritional support of essential minerals that have gone missing. As the body is cleansed, the mind clears. As the mind clears, the spirit lightens. As suggested earlier, now is the time to bear down and open the mind. Go slowly with new information so it can be easily digested. Though it may feel like going uphill, there is no rush. Pace yourself. Your mind will thank you on the downward slope when when you focus on the nature of the mind and spirit. So first, in order to appreciate the miracle of the body, lets "get physical."

THE BODY

Chapter Three

A BUG'S LIFE

The human body is a miracle of creation. Our bodies are made up of organ systems, interconnected through an array of bones, nerves, blood, lymph, and energy, all working in concert, each functioning cell representing a microcosm of the whole body. The first step in understanding the physical body is to go beyond the level of the organ system and acknowledge the most underappreciated aspect of our bodies, the microbe.

Of the hundred trillion cells that make up the body, roughly 100 trillion bacterial microbes inhabit our gut alone, consisting of about two pounds of weight. Our microbes also live on our skin, on the tongue, in our blood, and inside our cells. In fact, our microbes outnumber our human cells ten to one.[18] Their presence in the gut is the reason the gut makes up about ninety percent of our immune system. The immune system also includes the thymus, spleen, lymph, and mucous membranes of the body. In numbers, it is speculated that the adult human gut may contain up to 40,000 different bacterial species or nine million bacterial genes (compared to 20,000 human genes)[19] The sheer diversity of microbes illustrates the extent to which these bugs work to ensure their own survival. To date, only about one percent of human gut microbes have been identified.

The types of bacteria we host determine how we feel, how heavy or thin we are, how we age, and whether we are susceptible to illness or not. When our microbes are not happy, we feel it. When they are ill, so are we. Exactly which types of bacteria populate the gut determines how our immune system gets turned on or off.[20]

The beneficial bacteria that colonize our gut are the same bugs found in fertile soil. They are the same bugs found in fresh water. They live wherever you might imagine them - in the deepest layer of the earth's crust, in the low-temperature, high-pressure, reduced oxygen environment of a glacial core sample, and in the upper troposphere, ten kilometers above the Earth's surface. Knowing this we cannot deny our inherent connection to Nature. We come to understand that if we wish to sustain the human species, we must also sustain these microscopic species that live with us. We truly are what we eat, as well as what the plants and animals we consume eat. The root of our health really comes from the complex biodiversity of the soil where our food is grown.

Few people understand the "dirt" about microbes or what their presence might mean for overall physical well-being. Yet, sustainable, organic farmers have long known that the benefits of fertile, healthy soil come from the *life* found in the soil, known by science as homeostatic soil microorganisms. According to Jo Handelsman, professor of plant pathology at the University of Wisconsin, one gram of soil has potentially 100,000 species.[21] Like the human gut, it is nearly impossible to quantify the dimension of the unseen majority of microscopic life except to acknowledge that 99.9 percent of all microbes in the soil are still unknown.[22] Suffice to say that there are more bacteria in a handful of dirt than humans on the entire planet.

In our external environment, soil microorganisms not only recycle carbon and other soil nutrients from which plants develop. They are also responsible for purifying water, detoxifying harmful substances, and recycling waste products. They restore carbon dioxide to the air and make the atmosphere's nitrogen available to plants. Without them, continents would be deserts. All along the human digestive tract, these same microbes make up a highly organized micro-world, each species with its own vital function to maintain equilibrium. Some of their functions include:

- populate and reinforce a physical barrier.
- digest, ferment, and absorb nutrients from food.
- provide nutrients and energy (metabolism) for cells in GI tract.
- detoxify intestinal tract of opportunistic flora (parasites, viruses, fungus) by dissolving their cell membranes.

- neutralize and inactivate toxic substances and absorb carcinogenic substances.
- produce vitamins.[23]
- recruit immune cells to the site of infection and direct the body to produce the T-helper cells that seek and destroy pathogens that enter the body.

The world of the microbe is highly efficient. Nothing goes to waste, even the waste from beneficial bacteria helps control body weight by allowing your food to slow down so that nutrients can be absorbed.[24] If there is any one system that is the foundation of true health for the whole body, it is the digestive system. The more we know about our friendly bugs, the more they show themselves to be absolutely vital to both human health and the health of the planet. So it makes sense to understand the ideal conditions in which they live.

A Bug's Home

Our bugs make an ideal home in the mucous membranes of the immune system, which includes nose, mouth, as well as the millions of small, finger-like, tight folds called *villi*, located in the alkaline mucosal lining of the small intestine. Throughout the body, this one-layer mucosal surface is where our microbes protect the body against foreign substances and unfriendly bacteria, with the ability to neutralize them. The mucosal layer of the small intestine is also where some enzymes are produced for food digestion and absorption.

The 20-ft small intestine is part of the larger 25-foot intestinal tract considered to be immune "command central" for the body. This complex channel connects the esophagus to the anus, and provides a barrier between the outside world and our internal cells, between the food we eat and the blood that feeds our cells. It represents an ecosystem where our food is digested and absorbed and where it is transformed into microscopic particles that all of our cells use for energy, maintenance, and repair.

Once food is digested, food particles pass through the *villi* and into the bloodstream where they are incorporated into cells. At the same time that our blood receives filtered nutrient-rich molecules, our bugs, other larger molecules, and toxins are held back in the sanctuary of the small intestine. Other legions of defenses located here include:

GALT (gut-associated lymphatic tissues) – or mucosa-associated lymphoid tissue – Peyer's Patches, Secretory IgA, bacteriophages,[25] and macrophages. All stand ready to mobilize against any would-be foreign intruder. This is the reason this lining is said to comprise seventy percent of the immune system.[26]

We are born with bodies programmed to taste our surroundings, sense the environment, and protect us with a strong immune system. Recently, however, something has gone terribly wrong. GI disease and more severe, chronic diseases are now frequently diagnosed in children and adults alike. Common GI ailments such as constipation, reflux, abdominal pain, and inflammatory bowel disease have reached epidemic proportions in all age groups. Systemic inflammation throughout the body is manifesting in skin conditions (dermatitis herpetiformis), bone (oseteoporosis), infertility, and neurologic and psychiatric conditions (Alzheimer's and Parkinson's Disease). In the 1960s and 1970s, the subspecialties of pediatric gastroenterology and neurogastroenterology did not even exist. Today these fields are growing. Where did all of this disease begin?

The Antibiotic Revolution

In 1928, Alexander Fleming kicked off the antibiotic revolution with his discovery of Penicillin. Antibiotics were used successfully during World War II for wound infections and soon became standard issue in a world dominated by infectious disease. Yet the programmed fear of germs created ever newer and stronger antibiotics. In response, bacteria have resisted and gradually remade themselves into villains of the bug world – the superbugs. The antibiotic solution has created catastrophic problems, as reflected in the thousands of deaths each year from MRSA (Methicillin Resistant Staphylococcus Aureus), a drug-resistant and virulent mutant of the Staphylococcus aureus bacterium.

Antibiotics, whose name means "anti-life," are known to permanently alter gut bacteria. The antibiotic solution to the germ has killed off the good with the bad, creating the superbugs that have systematically dismantled our friendly microbial defenses. Such destruction, in combination with poor diet, has resulted in a nation left vulnerable to food allergies, recurrent infections, inflammation, immune dysfunction, and degenerative diseases.

We unknowingly participate in self-extermination when we fail to acknowledge our microbes, the heroes and anti-heroes that make us who we are. In any story the anti-hero is just as significant as the hero. They have a purpose and a role to fulfill. Though anti-heroes may come off as jerks, at their heart they must have heroic qualities – intrigue, sex appeal, strength – to be able to gain the sympathy of the audience; you. You must appreciate their role and what they have to offer in the larger picture. Once the anti-hero is acknowledged, he has the opportunity to turn himself around. The moral of the story is that most of today's diseases are greater than ninety percent preventable and reversible through a change in diet and lifestyle, and by recapturing knowledge and wisdom of the ages.

We can repopulate the body with beneficial bacteria with probiotics, meaning "for life," that come in the form of fermented foods (e.g., kefir, kombucha, kimchi). We have access to Nature's antimicrobials like raw honey, with its powerful enzymes known to destroy pathogens through its desert-like, moisture-sucking properties. We can utilize liquid iodine (the only beneficial halide) and liquid colloidal silver. Both iodine and silver selectively destroy the cell membrane of pathogens causing cell apoptosis (cell death). A testament to silver's healing properties is seen through its recent addition to antibiotics to increase effectiveness by up to 1,000 times against antibiotic resistance, even though the colloidal silver seems to be pulling all the weight.[27] In finding health we need only to remember the wisdom of Hippocrates and like-minded healers who came after. They showed that nutrition, together with each person's unique physique and sensibilities, are powerful tools in the healing arts.

The truest way to build health is to acknowledge that our bodies are complex ecosystems, dependent upon the connection between our macroenvironment and our microenvironment. Our friendly bacteria are critical companions in the delicate balance of our immune function. They are the gatekeepers to true health. The gut should reflect eighty-five percent friendly bacteria to fifteen percent unfriendly bacteria. The reverse of this ratio is called *dysbiosis* and characterizes the majority of people with chronic disease conditions. Without the right composition of gut bacteria, the energy balance from food changes to affect weight, age, and behavior.[28] [29]

Microbes, Weight, Age, and Behavior

Researchers finds that not only do bacteria affect the molecules inside the gut but they also influence our mood, feelings, and behavior, from how we react to stress to why we crave certain foods. What we eat not only affects the gut flora composition, but it can be argued that the composition of our gut flora affects the mind.

A 2013 Canadian study showed that connections between brain regions differed based on the species of bacteria that dominated the gut.[30] One species of microbe can select for anxious feelings while another can promote feelings of calm (i.e., gut feelings), showing that our microbes determine how brain circuits develop and how they are wired. Gut microbes seem to talk to the mind via the vegas nerve, the super highway that links gut to brain. Yet microbes also talk to the body in other ways, by modulating the immune system through production of custom versions of neurotransmitters, antibiotics, and chemicals that affect the nervous and endocrine systems, as well as all cells.[31]

Research from Emory University showed that the microbes we host partly determine our behavior and what we choose to eat.[32] For example, most people unbalanced in gut bacteria create acidic conditions in the body, meaning the overall pH of the cells and tissues (not the blood) is less than the ideal pH of 6.4. An acid environment invites bad bacteria, viruses, and yeast and fungus into the sanctuary of the small intestine and throws off equilibrium. With an increase in yeast and fungus, sugar cravings (and trips to the freezer for ice cream) are increased. In short order, a negative feedback loop can cause the accumulation of toxic waste products by a growing population of bad bacteria.

Our bacteria seem to be able to grow at different rates and control how long they live based on the conditions of their environment. Bacteria either seem to reproduce at high rates and lower yields, or at low rates (slow growing) and higher yields.[33] In nutrient-rich environments, bacteria with high growth rates are likely to be favored, whereas in nutrient-poor environments, slow-growing bacteria with higher biomass conversion efficiency is favored [34] Bacteria, like us, adapt to their surroundings in order to survive and age gracefully.

The importance of housing the right flora at an early age should not be underestimated. Flora is passed from mother to child in natural childbirth through the birth canal and with breastfeeding. The child also comes in contact with microorganisms from other family members. If the mother is overweight, the child can inherit "obese bacteria."[35] Evidence also suggests that children born via caesarean section have double the risk of becoming overweight according to researchers who found that differences in gut bacteria during the first year of life have been associated with higher risk of obesity later in life.[36]

However, antibiotics have immediate negative effects on weight. Antibiotics interfere with important hunger hormones secreted by the stomach and lead to increased appetite and body mass index (BMI).[37] Farmers have purposely used antibiotics in agriculture practices non therapeutically as growth promoters. Similarly, farmers use skim milk (not whole raw milk) to increase fat in pigs because removing the milk fat in the cream leaves only the milk sugar (lactose), which leads to weight gain. The same association was seen in a recent Harvard study of 12,829 children ages 9 to 14.[38] Those who drank more than three eight-ounce servings of low-fat milk a day gained the most weight, even after the researchers took into consideration factors such as physical activity, other dietary factors and growth. Compare pasteurized skim milk to whole fat "raw milk," a probiotic live food with beneficial bacteria and enzymes for complete digestion, and you see there are two different milks. Raw milk and its immune properties completely satisfies the appetite and prevents overeating.

Probiotics (e.g., raw milk) provide beneficial bacteria that have been widely used to improve intestinal balance in humans, farm animals, and pets.[39] So it would make intuitive sense that probiotics should be used in conjunction with antibiotics when prescribed by a medical doctor in order to help reestablish a healthy GI system. Simply adding a daily probiotic supplement to any diet with the species Lactobacillus and Bifidobacterium can help to maintain a healthy bodyweight and promote weight-loss.[40] [41]

Our gut environment plays numerous important roles, from maintaining stasis to affecting body weight and behavior, to how we age, to other roles for which we are only beginning to understand.[42] We are more than our genes. We are the food we eat and the microbes we maintain. We are the choices we make.

In her book *Why Dirt is Good,* Immunologist Mary Ruebush, Ph.D. writes, "What a child is doing when he puts things in his mouth is allowing his immune response to explore his environment ... the most delightful sights for a parent should be a young child covered in dirt from an active afternoon of outdoor play."[43]

If children are not exposed early in life to dirt, bugs, and bacteria, their bodies are not able to calibrate between harmless and harmful exposures. A 2006 study showed that unless children are exposed to a reasonable, full range of microbes in their natural environment, their immune systems may become hyper-sensitive and mount the inappropriate, excessive responses that lead to allergies, asthma, and inflammatory skin and bowel disorders.[44] [45]

Research focused on children raised on farms shows those exposed to a wide range of bugs possess strong allergy-protective properties that build the immune system.[46] A review of studies conducted worldwide in rural settings showed that the "farm effect," due to both inhaled (contact with livestock) and ingested (unprocessed milk from grass-fed cows) exposures, produced the most protective factors against allergies.[47] In 2006, the European PARSIFAL group published results of a five-year study of 15,000 children in five European countries and concluded farm milk consumption protected against asthma and allergy in rural and suburban populations across Europe. Additional research confirmed these results.[48] The greatest benefits came from drinking raw milk from grass-fed cows, full of beneficial bacteria.[49]

Even in light of these findings, modern society continues its aversion to dirt, as seen through the marketing of anti-bacterial soaps and wipes and irradiated, sterile, and processed foods. We only need to point to ourselves as the cause of the rise in asthma, allergies, autoimmune diseases, and cancer; the "diseases of civilization," as Thomas Cowan, M.D. describes in his book *Fourfold Path to Healing*.[50] Our high-tech focus on synthetic food and medicine finds us living in a germ-a-phobic world based on our collective, implicit belief that microbes are the enemy and the human body the victim.

Leaky Gut Syndrome

In living symbiotically with our natural environment, we are not victims of our own biology. So when all else fails, trust your gut. For your bugs to take care of you, you must take care of your gut. The thin mucosal lining of the gut is highly sensitive to irritants such as stress, prescription drugs (statins), environmental toxins (heavy metals), alcohol, and altered foods known as genetically modified organisms (GMOs), which comprise most of the western diet. When the intestinal lining becomes inflamed, it can tear, creating holes between the cells that are normally held tightly together.

A permeable or leaky gut means that several things are happening at once:

- The protective mucus is worn down, causing the alkaline pH of the gut to become acidic.
- Beneficial bacteria fail to thrive and cannot protect against opportunistic microbes that overgrow. Dysbiosis and yeast overgrowth result.
- The barrier system is breached so food particles and chemicals leak into the bloodstream.
- Toxic microbes produce toxins that flow through the damaged gut wall into the blood.
- An inflammatory alarm response is triggered throughout the whole body.

Leaky gut can begin with one course of antibiotics prescribed for a Strep infection. Conditions worsen when continuous antibiotic use fuels more infections. Next, a change in the internal pH of your digestive system slows the production of enzymes for efficient digestion. Undigested food particles pass through the intestines quickly without being absorbed. Oil-soluble hormones like thyroid replacement hormone, and vitamins D, A, E, and K are poorly absorbed which begins a cascade effect. Weight loss can result from malnutrition.[51]

A healthy source of fatty acids and cholesterol become essential for gut integrity and healing to be able to absorb fat-soluble vitamins. However, when a typical carbohydrate diet of pasta and bread is eaten, it further harms the body. Not only does the food not get digested and broken down, but it ferments and feeds the pathogenic bacteria and yeast in the gut to produce toxic products from its metabolism. In turn, the body craves more carbohydrates and sugars, which cause blood sugar levels to swing. Because white sugar burns up B-vitamins (for nerves, blood, etc.), chromium (for blood sugar balance), and calcium (for hormones and bones), nutrient deficiencies develop and symptoms begin.

Since each person is unique emotionally, mentally, and physically, there is no single cause for Leaky Gut Syndrome. Some of the most common causes and symptoms are:

Common Causes of Leaky Gut Syndrome:
· Air pollution (indoor and outdoor)
· Chronic stress/trauma (cortisol increases which increases gut permeability)
· Dysbiosis (more bad than good bacteria)
· Prolonged use of antibiotics
· Prolonged use of all medications (chemicals and heavy metals)
· Endotoxins (products of metabolism)
· Excitotoxins (MSG, additives, colorings)
· Chemotherapy/radiation
· Immune system overload
· Immunodeficiency of Secretory IgA
· Artificial sweeteners (Aspartame®)/artificial colors
· GMO foods (ninety-five percent of processed foods contain GMOs)
· Vegetable oils (soy, corn, canola)
· Alcohol overuse
· Chronic infections/presence of pathogens, parasites, yeast
· Refined/processed and microwaved foods

Common Symptoms of Leaky Gut Syndrome:

Aggressive behavior	Mood swings
Anxiety	Nervousness
Asthma	Poor exercise tolerance
Bed-wetting	Poor immunity
Chronic joint pain	Poor memory
Chronic muscle pain	Primary biliary cirrhosis
Confusion/fuzzy thinking	Recurrent bladder infections
Depression	Recurrent vaginal infections
Diarrhea	Recurrent strep throat infections
Fatigue and malaise	Shortness of breath
Fevers of unknown origin	Skin rashes/hives

Chapter Four

THE GERM VS. THE TERRAIN: A SHORT HISTORY

Since the Dark Ages, consensus has been split regarding the nature of disease and health. While disease-based medicine is built on the idea that a germ causes disease, many in the health field believe the strength of the immune system – the terrain – determines health. They believe the germ is merely the product of disease.

In modern times, western medicine popularized The Germ Theory of Disease defined by French chemist and biologist Louis Pasteur. Pasteur believed that germs attack the body from the outside to cause disease. His reasoning was based on his own experiments which showed that bad bacteria were responsible for souring wine and beer and could be removed by boiling and then cooling the liquid. This process was later extended to the milk industry as pasteurization in 1862. Pasteur went further to suggest that germs could be prevented through vaccination, a concept Edward Jenner postulated in 1796. Few voices at the time questioned Pasteur's theory or asked the question: if germs caused disease then why would some people get sick while others did not? Likewise, why did some people get well while others did not?

Two voices who disagreed strongly with Pasteur's ideas were his colleagues, Claude Bernard (1813-1878) and Antoine Bechamp (1816-1908). Both men viewed the body as a biological ecosystem in which nutritional status, toxicity, and pH were key factors. They considered germs to be the scavengers of disease that manifest when the body's natural metabolic processes are thrown off.

In his book *The Third Element of the Blood*, Bechamp identified a certain group of microbes that take on different forms, acting like shapeshifters based on the chemistry of their environment. Bad bacteria, viruses, and fungi, he argued, are merely the forms assumed by the bugs when the terrain favors disease. These bugs give off toxic byproducts, further contributing to a weakened terrain. According to Bechamp and Bernard, germs were merely symptoms, which lead to more symptoms to become a disease. It was no surprise that Bechamp soon became Pasteur's rival and argued against healing with vaccines, stating, "The most serious disorders may be provoked by the injection of living organisms into the blood."

Despite petty rivalries, the nineteenth century was a hotbed of natural healing opportunities. During this time, Sebastien Kneipp, Louis Kühne, and Dr Benjamin Lust inspired the birth of Neo-Naturopathy. Dr. Lust founded the American School of Naturopathy, the first college of its kind in the United States. These men followed Hippocrates's philosophy that "Nature is the physician of disease" and the physician's job is to help the healing process along, not to overtake it. They believed an inappropriate diet led to intestinal toxicity, which caused disease. In their view, naturopathy has only one purpose: to increase the vital force.[52]

> *"One of the first duties of a physician is the educate the masses not to take medicine.*

~*William Osler, M.D. "Father of Modern Medicine" (1849-1919)*

Another Hippocratic fan, Russian Nobel Laureate Elie Metchnikoff (1845-1916) also believed that "death begins in the colon." Based on his research in the 1900s, he forwarded the notion that the origin of all disease stems from the accumulation of waste matter and toxins in the body from constipation which weakens the terrain. Without a healthy elimination system, toxic by-products of the bowel bacteria are held in the body. Disease results when normal elimination functions fail to carry off the toxin and it enters the blood. Metchnikoff held that consuming beneficial lactic acid-producing bacteria found in fermented milk or yogurt as probiotics prevented growth of the unfriendly or putrefying bacteria.[53]

Others observed that fasting could heal elimination pathways by allowing body and mind to rest for a few days. Those who practiced naturopathy and homeopathy were critical of the suppressive nature of conventional drugs. They understood that masking a person's symptoms created deeper problems. They found that the fermentation of acids and alkaloids in the body, trapped in the colon, attracts germs in the same way that a garbage dump attracts flies that feed upon it. One study conducted at a government hospital attempted to prove the Germ Theory by injecting influenza germs into hundreds of patients. However, in each case, the onset of the disease did not appear. Others continued to challenge the Germ Theory.[54]

From the 1840s to the 1920s, natural physicians like Dr. Henry Lahn, MD (Iridologist), Sebastion Kneipp (Naturopath), and Samuel Hahnemann (Homeopath) all belonged to disciplines that enjoyed widespread popularity. It was Hahnemman (1755-1843), the founder of homeopathy, whose influence spread to the United States in the late 1800s from Germany. The success of homeopathic treatment for various endemic diseases like yellow fever and cholera was impressive. Death rates in homeopathic hospitals from these epidemics were often one-half to one-eighth those in orthodox medical hospitals where bloodletting, purging, and toxic chemicals were standard protocol.

By the early 1900s there were twenty-two homeopathic medical schools (e.g., Boston University, New York Medical School, Stanford University), 100 homeopathic hospitals and over 1,000 homeopathic pharmacies. In fact, homeopathy grew so quickly that in 1844 they organized the American Institute of Homeopathy – the first national medical society.[55] It was of no surprise that these forms of natural medicine created a growing opposition from establishment medicine not only for their healing successes but also because economic issues played a major role; the homeopathic hospitals got the business.

"Homeopathy cures a larger percentage of cases than any other method of treatment. Homeopathy is the latest and refined method of treating patients economically and non-violently."

~Mahatma Gandhi

In the area of disease prevention, the 1920s saw the innovations of Cleveland dentist Dr. Weston A. Price (1870-1948). Price traveled his own journey of health after the death of his son from a heart attack caused by a root canal procedure he performed. After visiting the most remote locations around the world, Price found that the healthiest cultures did not suffer tooth decay or any degenerative diseases, including cancer, due to a native, nutrient-dense diet and a lack of processed, refined foods (white sugar, flour). Dr. Price attributed tooth decay to: 1) not enough minerals in the diet; 2) not enough fat-soluble vitamins (A, D, E, and K) in the diet; and 3) inability of the intestinal system to absorb nutrients.

In the 1930's a healing ranch in California was opened by Naturopath Dr. Bernard Jensen, D.C. Ph.D. Jensen had healed himself of an incurable condition after having investigated all known natural modalities from nutrition to Herbology, Homeopathy, Heliotherapy, Hydrotherapy, Reflexology, Iridology, and many other drugless therapies. Jensen said, "We do not catch diseases, we create them by breaking down the natural defenses according to the way we eat, drink, think, and live. The germ exists only when the environment of the organism is favorable to its growth."[56]

German-born doctor Max Gerson, M.D.(1881-1959) emigrated to the United States and successfully treated many in the 1940s and 50s. Gerson innovated with his diet – The Gerson Therapy – using live and fresh green juices. After healing his own immune system, he helped others to reverse heart disease, kidney failure, arthritis, and many degenerative diseases, including cancer.

Outside the mainstream of medicine, more evidence reinforced the truth that germs seek their natural habitat – diseased tissue – and do not cause disease. Dr. Carey Reams (1903-1985), an agronomist, biochemist, physician, and mathematician (and friend of Einstein), showed that soil microbes, plants, animals, and humans each exist and function at a unique electrochemical frequency.

Reams understood the significance of Einstein's energy equation of taking things apart and showed through his own theory that things can be put back together. His Biological Ionization Theory is the study of how energy becomes matter and how matter becomes energy on a continuous basis." The loss of energy in humans is the start of disease.

Reams found that if the ionic mineral energy that flows through each species is not at its proper frequency then health and well-being naturally decline. He showed that nutrient mineral density of our foods directly impacts the quality of the digestive system, and that digestive integrity is absolutely required to maintain the electrochemical body "on frequency" for ideal health.[57]

Reams represented the last of a breed of natural healers that struggled against the tide of modern medicine. He devoted his life to helping thousands of people reverse tumors and other disease conditions. Based on his knowledge of plant health, he found that calcium is often the most crucial mineral in the human body for healing. Calcium, known as "the knitter" is transported by the blood to every cell of the body. The body requires more calcium by weight and volume than any other mineral. According to Reams, calcium is the best antioxidant in existence.[58]

"God is the basis of life, life is the basis of energy, energy is the basis of matter.

~Dr. Carey Reams

Reams discovery that a lack of calcium changes internal pH and leads to degenerative diseases has been systematically suppressed by drug research. Most people don't know that calcium is a multi-tasker: 1) it transfers signals among the endocrine glands and the nervous system; 2) it acts as a catalyst for many cell chemical activities including muscle contraction, and 3) it is necessary for nerve impulse transmission, thickness of cell membranes, strong bones and teeth, B12 absorption, and modulates the production of hormones. Using the pH of saliva and urine as a gauge, Reams showed how anyone can move the body into a healing range using various forms of calcium, lemon water, and distilled water, along with whole foods and lifestyle changes.

The Flexner Report

In the early 1900's the choices offered in natural healing were on the verge of a major shift. With the creation of the AMA in 1847, orthodox medicine sought to elevate medical education in order to improve their outcomes.[59] Other, unstated goals included eliminating its competition of homeopathy, naturopathy, and other natural healing tools.

In 1908, the AMA created the Carnegie Foundation as a gatekeeper of standards for medical schools. They hired Abraham Flexner, an educational theorist with no health or medical training. In 1910, working with data from the AMA, Flexner produced a report entitled, *Medical Education in the United States and Canada.* Over the next decade, medical schools published a curriculum focused on the basic sciences and added 4100 hours of education. The report served a pivotal role in creating a systematized education and structure.[60] It focused the role of State boards as a means of internal control. It set medicine on a path fueled by analytical thinking, published research, training, and education over the ethics, service, and art of healing.

The Flexner Report had a profound effect on the culture of medicine and healing over the next twenty years. It transformed the personal nature of medicine into a biomedical systems model with theoretical science and hands-on clinical training as the gold standard. Clinical research and productivity overtook compassion and commitment to patients. Under Flexner's persuasion American medicine sacrificed the doctor-patient relationship in favor of the pursuit of technical knowledge.[61]

The AMA, with the backing of financiers like John D. Rockefeller, also sought to standardize conventional medicine to reduce or eliminate natural medicine – naturopathy, homeopathy, osteopathy, chiropractic – and its tools, even though Rockefeller, himself, used homeopathy as his preferred healing modality and drank raw milk from his own herd. But Rockefeller, oil tycoon that he was, was first and foremost a motivated investor and needed to rid the competition from the medical playing field so that he could gain a monopoly in the drug and pharmaceutical industry.

The findings of the Flexner Report served to promote the public outcry needed to deny relevancy to holistic medicine that had, to this point, been mainstream. By the 1940s, tougher restrictions reduced the number of medical schools (including homeopathic medical schools) by fifty-four percent, as well as available doctors in rural areas.[62] Because the AMA only endorsed schools with a drug-based curriculum, lack of funding threw the holistic schools to the curb. New rules suppressed the use of Nature's tools like hemp, a plant containing cannabis oil with tremendous healing benefits. Big Pharma, the brain-child of John Rockefeller, was soon born.

In the beginning, the Flexner-model of medicine was instrumental in moving allopathic medicine out of the dark days of bloodletting and medical superstition and into science with experiential knowledge and skills. However, it also served to eliminate choice. Today, as science has evolved and awareness about the body's self-healing aspects has grown, little growth has occurred in medical education to parallel those changes.[63] Medicine is entangled in outdated requirements and core curriculum with long hours that are no longer relevant to our modern digital age where learning can be practiced long distance and outside institutions.

Ironically, Flexner had recognized that medical education had to be flexible and have the mandate to adapt to changing scientific, social, and economic circumstances, in order to evolve. His ideals should have supported the restructuring of medical education that is long overdue.

With today's governmental ties to the insurance industry, the monopoly of Big Pharma, and the political organization of the AMA, allopathic medicine has fallen further away from patient care. The words germ, drugs, vaccine, disease, cure, and epidemic are part of the lexicon based in a belief system that a "cure" can be found based on the cause – the germ. The Germ Theory remains the foundation of microbiology, general science, and medical science, as seen by our reliance on antibiotics and our growing dependence on vaccines, which are promoted as the main preventative tools in the war against the germ and "catching a disease." However, the development of vaccines has exploded beyond viruses to include non-infectious conditions such as allergies and behavioral addiction.

With the constant warnings of flu epidemics, the medical system instills fear in the public against a threat that exists outside of ourselves and over which we have little perceived control. Nature's laws teach that an epidemic merely reflects the collective landscape or culture of a group of people who have been exposed to the same environment, the same toxins, eaten the same food, and lived under the same conditions.

Through public awareness and demand for choice, there is now a resurgence of interest in natural modes of healing. Homeopathy is popular in Great Britain where the Royal family has utilized it since the 1830s.[64] It is well matched for rural areas where clinics are rare, and is especially effective for acute infectious diseases and chronic conditions. It is also cheaper than drugs.[65]

People are also scrutinizing their food choices for health. They want a relationship with their food and the farmer who grows it. Many are returning to Nature's whole, raw and organic foods, and are willing to pay more now to prevent the higher costs of disease later. They see the positive results of Hippocrates' tagline, "Let food be thy medicine and medicine be thy food." This message lives on in through the The Raw Food Institute which teaches the protocols of Ann Wigmore, a pioneer in the use of wheatgrass juice and Living Foods for detoxifying and healing the body, and through the Weston A. Price Foundation, founded by Sally Fallon, which provides support to small farmers and access to cutting-edge research, and sources of nutrient-dense, raw foods and raw milk for everyone who wants it.

"I asked the waiter, 'Is this milk fresh?' He said, 'Lady, three hours ago it was grass."

~Phyllis Diller

The demand for natural and holistic health options is rising in the United States. A 2011 government survey showed forty percent of the population uses some form of complimentary medicine, spending billions of dollars out-of-pocket.[66] Whether people are choosing holistic medicine because it aligns with their philosophy, expands their options, or because they can no longer afford conventional disease-management, the Germ Theory appears to be losing its potency. [67]

Chapter Five

VACCINE-NATION

In Nature, when an ecosystem operates in a state of harmony, it finds balance. There is no need for outside forces of protection because all internal systems are innately in tune with each other and with their environment. The human body is the same. Digestion, absorption, metabolism, elimination of nutrients, and protection against foreign invaders all happen in complete synchrony if the body has the right tools.

Today in medicine, acquired immunity through vaccination is strongly promoted as the primary tool of prevention to the exterior threat of the germ. The terrain's natural ability to self-regulate and heal is completely overlooked. Injecting antigens and potential pathogens, along with chemicals and metal adjuvants (stimulants) directly into the bloodstream to provoke an antibody response violates Nature's laws.

"In 1993, a high court judge in the UK decided that it was impossible to know the exact contents of vaccines and that science had no idea what the cocktail of chemicals contaminants and heavy metals contained in vaccines could do to the human body, or why they would work to prevent disease."

~The British Medical Journal, 1993

Natural Immunity

In natural (cell-mediated) immunity, the body blocks a toxin by its first line of defense, the skin. Evading the skin, the toxin meets up with the defenses of the respiratory system – coughing, sneezing, and fevers – for removal. The most resistant invaders are met by the gut-associated lymph system, equipped with vessels of lymph, tonsils, nodes, adenoids, spleen, and thymus. The gut-lymph system is where bacteriophages and white blood cells stand ready, immature lymphocytes become activated T cells specific to the antigen-invader, and cytokines are released. The body works to keep the toxin from the blood at all costs.

Artificial Immunity

The artificial (humoral) immunity of vaccination injects an antigen into the blood to provoke the body to create antibodies so next time the body sees the antigen, antibodies bind and neutralize it. Artificial immunity circumvents the body's natural, cell-mediated pathways to provide a free pass straight to the blood where antigens can be transported anywhere in the body. The legions of defenses that would normally be called to duty end up sleeping on the job. Artificially provoking the immune system with vaccine ingredients that often resemble self – viral and bacterial DNA, proteins, adjuvants – can lead to different responses (e.g., cytokine releases) in different people, causing both allergic reactions,[68] autoimmune reactions,[69] [70] [71] [72] and leukemias.[73]

Not surprisingly, the logic and ritual behind mass vaccine campaigns by the Centers for Disease Control and Prevention (CDC) has not proved to be the advertised cure-all at all. The CDC's own numbers show that vaccines provoke the very diseases they claim to prevent. From the mid-1800s to the 1950s, up to eighty percent of those vaccinated against smallpox in India, England, and the United States contracted the disease.[74] In the 1960s, Americans continued to experience serious adverse events to the small pox vaccine, including death, post vaccine encephalitis, among other reactions.[75]

Polio Epidemic

In similar fashion, cases of paralytic polio continued after the initial Salk vaccination campaign in 1955.[76, 77] (See figure 1). Paralysis most often began at the site of injection. Similar reports were made in Canada, England, Holland, Austria, Germany,[78] Australia, Czechoslovakia, and in India.[79]

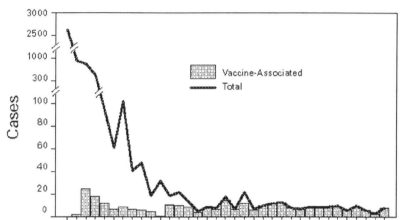

FIGURE 1. Total number of reported paralytic poliomyelitis cases* and number of reported vaccine-associated cases — United States, 1960–1994

*Excluding imported cases.

Figure 1

In an elaborate study conducted by the New York State Health Department during the polio epidemic of 1949 in the United States "contraction of polio by definite contact with other victims of the disease was not established."[80] However, there was an investigation of a possible link between cases of paralysis and Wyeth Laboratory, the lab that created the vaccine. Two reports that were not reported to the public concluded: "Some of these cases were known to be "vaccine associated.[81] [82]

In 1992, the CDC finally published a report admitting the polio vaccine was the cause of the disease, the reason it was pulled from the market.[83] Since the new inactivated vaccine was introduced, the warning remains that the vaccine can cause "serious problems and death."[84] [85]

The CDC claims that polio has been eradicated in the world. However, an increased incidence of vaccine-induced paralysis is causing many to wonder if polio has simply been renamed "non-polio Acute Flaccid Paralysis (AFP), "aseptic meningitis (Fields Virology), and Guillain-Barré Syndrome (GBS), a vaccine-induced disease.[86] [87] The symptoms between polio, AFP, and GBS are identical and include fever, headache, sore throat, vomiting, stiff neck and back, muscle weakness, pain in joints, and paralysis of one or more limbs or respiratory muscles.[88] Figure 2 shows the rise of AFP between 1996 and 2010 to coincide with the fall of polio (along bottom of graph).

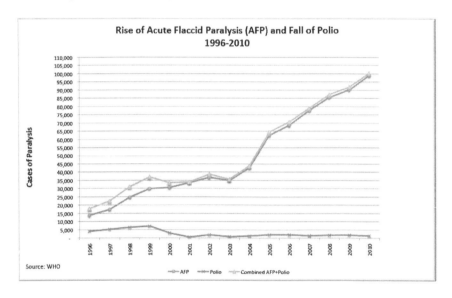

Figure 2 Credit: vaccinecouncil.org

India has not reported any wild polio for more than two years, however many areas are now reporting high numbers of AFP.[89]

> *"While it is possible that the surveillance system is so good that there is some amount of over-reporting, it is equally possible that some of these huge numbers of AFPs could be explained if we take into account the possibility of vaccine-derived polio cases. A 1700% rise or a 2300% rise cannot be otherwise explained."*
>
> *~ Dr Jacob Puliyel, Indian Journal of Medical Ethics, Apr-Jun 2012*

The subtle transition from infectious disease to vaccine-induced disease begs the question, does polio result from a living virus or from something else?

The 1940 medical dictionary defines the term *virus* as a poison. Poliomyelitis is from the Greek language, *polios* meaning gray, *myelos* meaning marrow, and *itis* meaning inflammation. In the 1940s during World War II and into the early 1950s massive amounts of poisons in the form of pesticides, DDT, malathion, heptachlor, dieldrin, TEPP were sprayed on crops and eaten by livestock and people, which were found to increase viral infections.[90] Some of the same chemicals used to spray pesticides (Tween 20, Tween 80, Triton X-100, Nonoxyenol-9) are still present in childhood vaccines.[91] [92] As DDT and other pesticides were phased out, cases of polio also began to decline. Note the strong association between the spraying of pesticides and the worst polio epidemic in United States history.

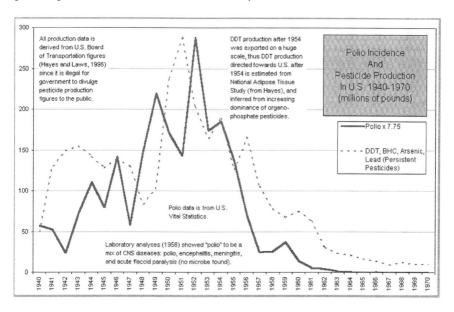

Figure 3

Focusing on the germ causation theory at the expense of all evidence not only leaves disease unchecked to spread, but it directs attention away from the real causes and meaningful investigation. Other conflicting factors included the recommendation of tonsillectomy during the polio epidemic which, ironically, often caused the worst kind of paralysis (Bulbar Poliomyelitis).[93] [94] [95] Do debilitating symptoms and deaths from vaccines continue based on a false theory of "catching a disease?"

Diet, Depletion, and Disease

The efficacy for vaccination has not been proven. Yet research clearly shows that multiple vaccinations can lead to a suppressed immune system,[96] and that diet plays a significant role. Vaccine toxicity plus a poor diet add up to disaster.

Vaccines cause the body to use up its vitamin stores to increase antibody production. Polio is almost identical to vitamin B1 deficiency (Beri Beri) from a nutrient-poor diet.[97] Refined (white) flour lacks many minerals and contains less than half the calcium, and a third the phosphorous and potassium. In 1952, Dr. Benjamin Sandler, M.D. warned people in North Carolina to stop eating ice cream and soda and subsequently saw the incidence of polio drop by ninety percent.[98] Patients who raised calcium levels to two-and-a-half times that of phosphorus saw degenerative diseases disappear. The prime culprits that cause an imbalance in the phosphorus calcium ratio are meat, sugar, and soft drinks.[99] Vitamin C was found to successfully treat acute poliomyelitis.[100]

Excess antibodies from vaccines cause the body to become hypersensitive which can bring about allergies and autoimmune conditions. Allergies represent the body's natural reaction to toxins in attempts to cleanse itself. This happens when the glands – the pancreas, pituitary, and spleen – become over-stimulated and reduce the body's ability to self-regulate.

Steroidal inhalers (albuterol) used to treat asthma stimulate the adrenal medulla of the brain where adrenalin and noradrenalin are made. These drugs stimulate the adrenals (not the lungs) due to adrenal exhaustion from toxins or stress. The adrenal glands and the pancreas work together to maintain a balanced blood sugar. So if the adrenal glands fail to function well, then blood sugar is a problem too. When the adrenals become overstimulated there is a decrease in circulation of blood throughout the body and the subsequent atrophy of vascular vessels.[101]

Pharmaceutical companies like Merck acknowledge the effects of their vaccines on the vaccine package inserts. "Cases of HIB disease, although rare, may occur after vaccination." Among those in the medical community, this reaction is known as 'Provocation Disease.' But what about Provocation Death? A document leaked to the public revealed that between 2009 and 2011 the new 6-in-1 Infanrix hexa vaccine by GlaxoSmithKline for babies resulted in at least seventy-three deaths and thousands of reports of adverse reactions.[102]

Officially, only one to ten percent of adverse vaccine events are ever reported to the Vaccine Adverse Reporting System (VAERS), a database overseen by the CDC and FDA.[103] Ninety percent go unreported.[104] The flawed system lacks traceability of safety, efficacy, and immunity. Of the 8,000 different adverse vaccine reactions listed, reports of life-threatening vaccine reactions (convulsions, anaphylaxis, SIDS, meningitis, encephalitis, autism, cardiac and respiratory arrest, pneumonia, etc.,) are more numerous than reported deaths. Permanent disabilities outnumber life-threatening reactions.

Ironically, pharmaceutical companies are completely immune from lawsuits in the marketplace thanks to the National Childhood Vaccine injury Act (NCVIA) Congress passed in 1986. The act states: "no vaccine manufacturer shall be liable...if the injury or death resulted from side effects that were unavoidable even though the vaccine was properly prepared and was accompanied by proper directions and warnings."

And yet, the toxic and experimental nature of vaccines is reflected by CDC's acknowledgment that the polio vaccine was dispensed knowing it contained the monkey virus SV40 shown to cause cancer in humans from the data of Italian researcher Michael Carbone in 1994.[105] These findings are linked to the administration of SV40-contaminated polio vaccines from 1954 until 1963.[106] In 2002, the *Journal Lancet* published evidence that contaminated polio vaccine is responsible for 55,000 non-Hodgkin's lymphoma cases each year.[107]

New Vaccines

A vaccine against malaria has remained an elusive goal for years due to the many strains of the parasite that transmits the illness known mainly in India and sub-Saharan Africa. Recently, the National Institutes of

Health (NIH) claims to have developed a safe malaria vaccine ready for approval.[108] However, the vaccine is less than fifty percent effective[109] and produces more virulent strains that cause worse symptoms in unvaccinated animal models.[110]

Perhaps the CDC's biggest question mark for the claim of vaccine "prevention" lies in its promotion of the annual flu shot since officials have to guess which viral strains will dominate in a given year. The flu vaccine is hyped to make us fear a mild condition that naturally cycles in greater than ninety-nine percent of the population. Tragically, serious injuries related to flu shots are growing more common each year while studies show the vaccine to be ineffective:

- In the aftermath of the 2009/2010 swine flu scare, children in England and throughout the world given the Pandemrix flu vaccine had a 1,400 percent increased risk of developing narcolepsy compared to those not vaccinated.[111] [112]
- The CDC reported that the 2009/2010 H1N1 flu shot in pregnant women, led to a 25-fold increase in incidence of of spontaneous abortion and miscarriages.[113]
- A 2011 study in the *International Journal of Medicine* revealed flu shots result in inflammatory cardiovascular changes indicative of increased risk for serious heart-related events such as heart attack.[114]
- According to a 2012 double-blind, randomized, controlled trial (the first of its kind) conducted in healthy children 6 to 15 years of age, getting a flu shot was found to increase the risk of other respiratory viral infections over four-fold.[115]
- A February 2013 report by the CDC found the flu shot only nine percent effective for seniors against the 2012-13 flu bug. Further, small children inoculated gained no protection from the disease.[116]
- The presence of adjuvants (aluminum) in the flu shot characterizes the classical antiphospholipid syndrome (APS) or 'Hughes Syndrome' by the presence of antiphospholipid antibodies (aPL). Through molecular mimicry, these antibodies bind negatively-charged phospholipids, platelets, and endothelial cells which affects multiple organs including heart, CNS, kidney, and skin.[117] [118]

In a recent report in the *British Medical Journal,* Peter Doshi, PhD of Johns Hopkins, charged that the flu shot is not only ineffective but the threat of the influenza virus is highly overstated because most people never actually end up contracting it. Through a misinformation campaign based in semantics, Doshi says influenza cases and flu/pneumonia cases are purposely lumped together even though "influenza" and "flu (or pneumonia)" are two different animals. In eighty-four percent of flu cases, no influenza virus is ever found based on sampling.[119]

In reality, populations are not sampled during flu season to determine which virus is actually circulating, let alone if it is viral or bacterial. In 2003, total deaths from the influenza virus were found to be 18, not the "36,000 annual flu deaths" publicized by the CDC and the media. Doshi says` most flu is really bacterial or fungal in nature, resulting from pollution and tainted foods – not viral. This means that even the most well matched flu vaccine to a wild influenza virus only targets a small part (sixteen percent) of those with flu.

In what should be front page headlines, the 2010 Cochrane Review – a systems review of primary research in human health care and health policy – found no evidence that flu vaccines affect complications, such as pneumonia, hospitalization transmission of flu between people, or death.[120] The review also found that studies funded from public sources were significantly less likely to report conclusions favorable to the vaccines while in the majority of industry-funded studies there was "evidence of widespread manipulation of conclusions and spurious notoriety of the studies." Claims that the flu vaccine cuts elderly deaths in half were negated: "Due to poor quality data of the available evidence any conclusions regarding the effects of influenza vaccines for people aged 65 years or older cannot be drawn."

> *"There are not enough influenza-related deaths to support the conclusion that vaccination can reduce total winter mortality among the U.S. elderly population by as much as half."*
>
> ~*Simonsen et al. Arch Intern Med. 2005; 165(3)*

In light of recent forced flu vaccines for medical staff, an open 2013 letter was published in the *Journal of American Physicians and Surgeons* questioning whether such mandates are medically warranted and ethically correct citing that the flu vaccine: 1) is a "statistical gamble" in targeting actual circulating viruses; 2) shows seventy percent of people are already immune at the time of vaccination, according to FDA studies; and 3) shows no evidence that it affects complications of pneumonia or transmission from person to person (as advertised).[121]

The truth about vaccines has also been surfacing in our children through increased outbreaks of mumps[122] [123] measles,[124] [125]and pertussis[126] [127] in *vaccinated* children. Recent evidence shows that vaccines are triggering more virulent microbes. The Chicken Pox vaccine is responsible for triggering a nationwide Shingles epidemic.[128] Vaccine-induced atypical measles is more serious than the "wild" measles virus. In both cases, the vaccine suppresses a child's rash, which is the body's natural pathway to excrete toxins. Instead, toxins are pushed deeper into the body to affect the major organs and sometimes the brain, as atypical measles encephalitis. Vaccine viruses can attach themselves to cells, organs and brain tissue and cause disabilities and brain injury, as in the case of a 13-year-old autistic boy. [129]

Not surprisingly, viruses and bacteria appear to have as much resistance to death as we do. By their very nature, they are built to survive and thrive. It is increasingly apparent that vaccine-related outbreaks are reflective of false claims about the efficacy of vaccines. Such is the case in the complaint against Merck's mumps vaccine, found to be based on sham testing.[130] Testing of the vaccine never included real mumps viruses yet claimed a "95% efficacy rate" based on blood tests that were artificially spiked with animal antibodies to inflate the appearance of immune system antibodies.[131] This fraud has been ongoing since the late 1990s so that Merck could maintain a monopoly in the market.

The real tragedy of vaccine-induced diseases goes beyond greed. They are causing harm to whole generations because these virulent forms manifest as more severe, chronic conditions than the naturally occurring viruses.

The Pertussis Vaccine Epidemic

We are not necessarily aware our microbes live with us until their actions show up as symptoms we resist. We are told to immunize so we don't end up with the bacterium that causes croup, and soon after we begin to experience asthma with every cold and flu that comes our way.

Several epidemiological studies show there is a much greater incidence of atopic disorders – asthma, eczema, ear infections – in fully vaccinated children as compared to those with limited or no vaccines.[132] [133] [134] [135] Children vaccinated against the bacterium that causes whooping cough are seventy-five percent more likely to develop asthma, hayfever, and eczema later in life.[136]

Like the flu, pertussis is a mild condition in otherwise healthy adults and children over two months. Symptoms include a cough, fever, and barking spasms but leaves no permanent damage. Mothers who had pertussis as children naturally pass on immunity to their children, which is protective during the first year along with breastfeeding. However, immunity from the vaccine may last only a few years if at all. The pertussis vaccine does not produce IgA, IgG, or IgM protective antibodies. It does, however, produce IgE antibodies associated with allergic disease. Only the natural infection with pertussis produces IgG, IgM, and IgA.[137]

Evidence of a worldwide increase in whooping cough and its death rate came from a 2005 study showing the organism B. pertussis mutated to a resistant form, B. parapertussis.[138] In Japan, tracking research after 1976 showed that as vaccine compliance for the pertussis vaccine began to climb so did the incidence of whooping cough, basically showing the vaccine to be irrelevant to the condition.[139] In England, despite vaccination rates of ninety-four percent in children under two, the incidence of pertussis has been increasing since 1995.[140] By 1992, the number of cases had already reached pre-vaccine levels. A 2013 study published in the *Journal Proceedings of the National Academy of Sciences*[141] concluded the efficacy of the acellular pertussis vaccines (DTaP) wanes after five years, and that those vaccinated become asymptomatic carriers to spread the infection to those who are unvaccinated.[142]

Pertussis Vaccine Side Effects

The pertussis vaccine is reported to bring on neurological complications, from convulsions to mental retardation and death,[143] and has provoked an increase in a bacterial infection Haemopilus influenzae type b (Hib),[144] and other bacterial illnesses. Hib can manifest as pneumonia, or cellulitis, arthritis, middle ear infection, osteomyelitis, conjunctivitis, respiratory infections, or none of them, depending on what is found in the laboratory. There is no clinical definition for this condition because Hib can be any disease with any symptoms. The Hib vaccine was introduced to combat an illness with no known source other than invasive bacterial infections, and without a way to properly monitor the vaccine's effectiveness. Yet the vaccine program claims to be able to track the effectiveness of vaccines in order to reduce disease rates and promote wellness. It is not widely publicized that cases of pertussis continue to peak every three to four years as part of a natural cyclical phenomenon in human populations.[145]

Pertussis-Diabetes Link

Published data in the medical literature suggests that not only diet, but the increasing number of childhood vaccines, may play a role in the big jump in the number of cases of juvenile diabetes. The pertussis toxin is a known trigger of juvenile diabetes as it affects the pancreas in its insulin-secreting parts. As early as the 1970s, the pertussis vaccine was documented to stimulate overproduction of insulin by the pancreas followed by exhaustion and destruction of the islets of Langerhans, resulting in diabetes.[146]

Between 1988 and 1991, there was a reported sixty percent increase in Type 1 diabetes following a massive campaign in New Zealand to vaccinate babies six weeks of age or older with hepatitis B vaccine.[147] Since 1996, evidence of a vaccination-diabetes connection has been strengthened by the epidemiological investigation of J. Barthelow Classen, MD, a former researcher at the National Institutes of Health who found that vaccines given to children at two months and older can induce immune-mediated diabetes.[148] He estimated over 10,000 cases of diabetes each year in the United States are vaccine-induced.[149, 150]

Homeopathic treatment is an option that can bring significant relief and shorten duration based on choosing a remedy that most closely matches the symptom profile. Though homeopathic medicine is FDA-approved and available over the counter, it is advisable to consult with a homeopathic professional due to the seriousness of the condition.

Inject to Protect

Vaccines are sold as a prevention for "the herd" against the few who are not "protected," even though whole civilizations have been raised without vaccines. Based on trends seen in diverse populations, "herd immunity" may be just another theory. In the case of pertussis, the mutated virus is not silenced but transformed.[151] Both strains of pertussis are seen in around the world and appear to have similar virulence, negating the effectiveness of the vaccine.[152]

The logic to require mandatory vaccination based on "herd immunity" is breaking down with each new outbreak in vaccinated herds. Mandatory vaccination is an assault on informed choice, personal freedom, and the body's immune system. Each DTaP shot contains aluminum formaldehyde, bovine protein, and polysorbate 80, an additive linked to GI problems, heart attacks, strokes, impaired immunity, and tumor growth. The CDC continues to recommend five doses of the DTaP shot for children in light of evidence that the vaccine may cause pertussis. Those who choose not to vaccinate their children should not anger those who choose to vaccinate. After all, if the vaccines work, why would a vaccinated child be at risk?

Vaccines vs. Clean Water

According to an editorial in the 1999 *Journal of Pediatrics*, "the largest historical decrease in morbidity and mortality caused by infectious disease was experienced not with modern anti-biotics and vaccines, but after the introduction of clean water and effective sewer systems."[153]

In the 2002, the *Journal Lancet Infectious Diseases* graphically made this point. Using raw data from the 1900s, overall mortality from infectious disease had declined to negligible levels long before the introduction of widespread vaccination practices.[154] Figure 4 comes from the 1937 "Vital Statistics of the United States."[155]

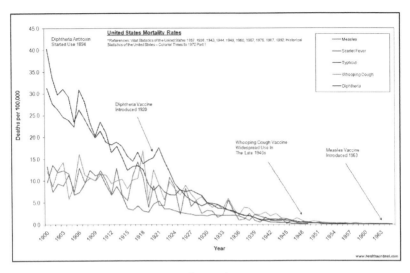

Figure 4

A 2012 Polish report describes that despite the claim for the need of immunization, there are now strong reasons to argue against it.[156] To illustrate this, figure 5 shows the pertussis (whooping cough) mortality rate from 1838 to 1976 in England/Wales revealed the death rate from pertussis maintained the same downward trend before and after the time vaccines were implemented.

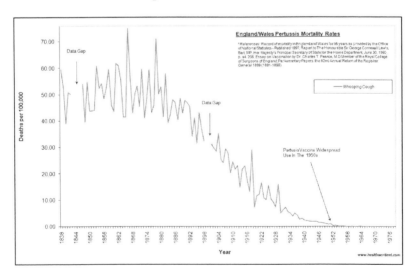

Figure 5

Similarly, Figure 6 shows the number of all infectious deaths in England had been in a steady decline before the small pox, diphtheria, pertussis, and measles vaccines were introduced, and they maintained the same downward slope thereafter.

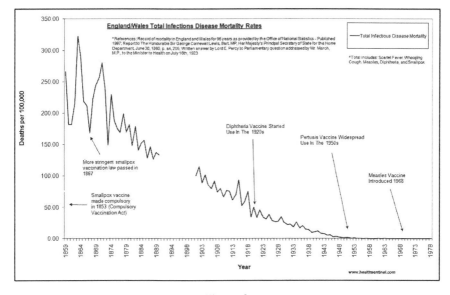

Figure 6

The idea of vaccines had originally been based on the first law of homeopathy of 'like-cures-like" in exposing the body to a minute amount of substance that causes symptoms of the disease in order to stimulate an immune response for the body to heal itself. Yet where homeopathy uses a "nosode," a substance that is serially diluted in purified water and shaken until only the harmless essence remains to promote healing on an energetic level, allopathic medicine uses the whole antigen, live or dead, with added toxins to artificially stimulate the body into producing an antibody response in acquired – or artificial – immunity.

Vaccines have become profit-generating, bio-engineered products increasingly mandated by government. The shots contain elements unnatural to the body – heavy metals, carcinogens such as phenol, formaldehyde, polysorbate 80, antibiotics, aluminum salts, latex rubber, genetically modified yeast, human cells, foreign animal and cancer related proteins, viral and bacterial DNA, microorganisms, monosodium glutamate, mercury, and gelatin from cattle and pigs.[157] These ingredients – banned in food products and soft drinks (except formaldehyde) – are all listed on the package insert that anyone can request.

The authors of the Polish study point out the concern by doctors over the decline of children's health since the 1960s, which coincided with increased vaccinations. The study identified two main categories of adverse effects following vaccination: 1) early post-vaccine complication, and 2) late and long-term complications affecting the nervous system. They noted that anaphylactic reaction occurs most often after immunization against typhoid, tetanus, pertussis, measles, mumps, and rubella.

Immediate Reaction	Central Nervous System Reactions
Redness	Encephalopathy
Swelling	Febrile convulsions
Pain	Non-febrile convulsions
Lymphadenopathy	Paralytic *poliomyelitis* caused by vaccine virus
Muscle pain	Encephalitis
Joint pain	Meningitis
Flu-like symptoms	Gullian-Barré syndrome

Vaccine Schedule

American children today receive 49 doses of fourteen different viral and bacterial vaccines before age six.[158] The CDC vaccine schedule recommends thirteen shots in the first year and twenty shots within the first two years of life. Compare these numbers to Japan's where 6 shots are recommended in the first year and only three in the second year of life. In 1975, Japan raised its minimum vaccination age to two years and saw a subsequent drop in overall infant mortality rate, which in 1975, was noted to be the lowest in world rankings.[159] However, while infant mortality rates fell from 1975 to 1976 due to non-compliance, rates began to rise again between 1976 and 1979 when compliance increased with new parents who did not have previous information and populations with short attention spans. In Japan, low compliance seemed to be linked to low death rate and vise versa.[160]

The CDC's recommended childhood immunization schedule requires infants to receive up to eight vaccines simultaneously affecting millions of infants each year and without ever having been formally tested. In a 2012 peer-reviewed study, researchers found babies who received the most vaccines (three or more at the same time) tended to have higher hospitalization and death rates. In fact, "hospitalization rate increased linearly from 11.0% for infants receiving 2 vaccine doses to 23.5% for infants receiving 8 vaccine doses." [161]

> *"A single vaccine given to a six-pound newborn is the equivalent of giving a 180-pound adult 30 vaccination on the same day."*
>
> *~Dr. Boyd, Toxicologist, retire professor of Chemistry, University of Kentucky*

Seeing similar trends, Japan, in 1993, discontinued the bundled MMR vaccine and reverted to three separate injections for mumps, measles, and rubella. The MMR vaccine had been linked to outbreaks of non-viral meningitis, other damaging side effects, and deadly epidemics from measles. Japan has since discontinued compulsory vaccination of any kind.[162]

Vaccination is Not Immunization

Vaccine outbreaks in highly vaccinated populations are showing that vaccination is not immunization. Heavy metals like mercury and aluminum are neurotoxins that primarily settle in the brain. Ethyl mercury (thimerosal) was originally added to vaccines as a preservative and had been slated for removal from vaccines by 2001 due to the risks for neurotoxicity. But in fact, thimerosal still exists in most vaccines at 25mcg per dose, with young children often receiving five or more – bundled – vaccines in one visit. The 1978 Schubert study found that the amount of lead and mercury when each was given separately – lethal to one percent of rats tested – would become lethal for one hundred percent of rats tested when combined.[163] New research shows mercury to be toxic to mitochondria, shutting down the energy storehouse of cells.[164] Our mitochondria carry the descendants of the first bacteria from the oceans that learned to use oxygen. They now form a symbiotic relationship with our cells, providing energy in exchange for food and shelter.

"It is universally recognized among toxicologists that combinations of toxic chemicals may bring exponential increases in toxicity; that is, two toxic chemicals in combination will bring a ten-fold or even a hundred-fold increase in toxicity."

~Dr. Harold Buttram[102]

In preempting the body's natural processes through vaccination, we wage war on our bacteria. In our ignorance we have traded natural infectious conditions for chronic autoimmune disease. Germany released an independent survey in September 2011 of 8,000 unvaccinated children, newborn to nineteen years, which showed vaccinated children have at least two to five times more diseases and disorders than unvaccinated children.[165] A 2013 pediatric survey published in JAMA reported undervaccinated children, due to parental choice, had significantly fewer ER and outpatient visits over children who were vaccinated on schedule.[166] Currently, an independent study is underway in the United States comparing unvaccinated home-schooled children vs. vaccinated children to determine whether vaccinations are associated with long-term illness.[167] Ignorance is not bliss.

Adjuvants

Since the alleged mercury phaseout of thimerosal, another neurotoxin, aluminum "Alum" has been added as a main adjuvant. Adjuvants hyperstimulate the immune system to increase antibody titers using less antigen. Increased antibodies leads to increased inflammation. Using adjuvants like aluminum, or squalene (MF59) commonly used in the military, the immune system becomes supercharged but with no guarantee that the antibody will target the correct antigen. Evidence shows adjuvants induce ASIA (autoimmune syndrome induced by adjuvants)[168] which can manifest as encephalitis, chronic fatigue syndrome, macrophagic myofasciitis, subcutaneous pseudolymphoma, and siliconosis.[169, 170] A recent Canadian study showed that rates of autism increased during a seventeen-year period in countries where the majority of vaccines contained the adjuvant aluminum [171]. Strong evidence also shows that squalene may be directly responsible for triggering an epidemic of Gulf War Syndrome.[172] As with mercury, no studies exist to show how squalene or aluminum benefit health or if they are safe.

"Folks that fought alongside us in the Gulf War who did not take the anthrax vaccine have no incidence of Gulf War illness."[121]

~Capt. Rovet, RN, BSN, B-C (USAF ret).

What is known is that, according to a CDC epidemiologist,[173] aluminum accumulates in the skin, blood, bones, and brain and data shows significant associations between aluminum and mercury and neuro-developmental delays. A 2011 study in the *Journal of Inorganic Biochemistry* showed a strong correlation between aluminum vaccines and autism spectrum disorders (ASD). A 2011 report in the *Journal of Tropical Medicine* suggests a link between DTaP vaccines used in third world countries and Sudden Infant Death Syndrome.[174] Studies also confirm that the brains from Alzheimer's patients contain about 1.4 times the aluminum level found in those without Alzheimer's.[175]

The new tetanus-alum vaccine causes an autoimmune condition known both as Hughes syndrome and as Antiphospholipid Syndrome (APS). The mechanism involves molecular mimicry. Since these alum antigens are identical in makeup to phospholipids which form the cell membrane in every cell, they can attack any part of the body – the eye, cardiovascular system, brain, nerves, skin, reproductive system – but they are becoming known for causing heart attacks and fetal death.[176]

Vaccines with Human DNA

Helen Ratajczak, author of "Theoretical aspects of autism: Causes – A review" writes that when vaccine makers removed much of the mercury they replaced it with human tissue, which is currently used in twenty-three vaccines. She believes that the rise in autism may correlate to the introduction of human DNA in the MMR vaccine. Human DNA can potentially cause brain damage because the foreign DNA is incorporated into the host DNA which the body, seeing an altered self, attacks the neurons in the brain. While critics claim there is no proof that human DNA in vaccines causes autism, they ignore an established link to encephalopathy. Furthermore, there is no proof to the contrary – that human DNA in vaccines does not cause autism.

Guard Against Gardasil

With the vaccine market for infectious disease nearly saturated, new vaccines for non-infectious conditions such as autism,[177] cancer, and Alzheimer's using experimental genetic engineering are next. An example is Merck & Co.'s Gardasil vaccine, which targets four strains (out of one hundred plus) of the sexually transmittable Human Papillomavirus (HPV) said to cause cervical cancer. The HPV vaccine, marketed to young girls and boys age nine to fifteen, is only guaranteed effective for five years, well before this target group is sexually active. The vaccine contains fetal cell lines and genetically engineered human albumin, according to the insert.[178] Recently, one hundred percent of Gardasil samples tested were contaminated with residual viral DNA and RNA fragments.[179] These fragments were attached to Merck's proprietary aluminum adjuvant in one hundred percent of samples.

Foreign DNA fragments incorporate into the human genome to cause blood problems, joint pain, weakness, chronic fatigue, Guillain-Barré syndrome, fainting, seizures, lupus, blood clots, obesity, heart disease, diabetes, autoimmune diseases, Idiopathic Thrombocytopenia Purpura, a blood disorder that causes abnormal bleeding, brain inflammation, premature menopause in teens due to ovarian failure, and tumors.[180, 181, 182] There have been at least 140 deaths associated with this vaccine, and thousands of disabling injuries even as its promotion goes on.

Without follow-up protocols in place or informed-consent, parents are left in the dark about serious side-effects. It is also not disclosed to patients that: 1) cervical cancer risk is extremely low; 2) vaccines are unlikely to affect the rate of cervical cancer in the United States; 3) eight out of 10 sexually active women will have HPV in their life with no symptoms, and that greater than 98 percent of these clear themselves; 4) 70 percent of HPV infections naturally resolve themselves within a year; and 5) 90 percent of infections resolve within two years.[183] Japan's health ministry in 2013 issued a nationwide warning that the HPV vaccines are no longer recommended for girls aged twelve to sixteen due to several adverse reactions.

It appears that artificial immunity is based on the flawed pre 1940s ideas that antibody production from toxins equates to immunity. The true complexity of the immune system is more than just the simplified antibody mechanism artificially triggered by heavy metal stimulants and adjuvants.

Research in 2012 published in the *Journal Immunity* by Cell Press, shows that antibodies do not act alone to fight off infection. High levels of antibodies (humoral immunity) did *not*, in themselves, always ensure survival. The essential and true components are the B cells, the cells from which antibodies come, since they produce a chemical needed to maintain innate immune cells called macrophages. The macrophages produce type 1 interferons, which are required to prevent fatal viral invasion. Macrophages that defend against viruses are much like our non-host derived bacteriophages that defend against microbes, also without the aid of antibodies.[184] . Our mucus layer creates a reserve of bacteriophages extensive enough to protect against all the bacterial diseases encountering it.[185] Together it is our B cells and bacteriophages (cell-mediated mechanisms) that embody innate immunity, not our antibodies alone. This fact essentially nullifies the theory that vaccine-induced antibodies are required or serve any legitimate function in preventing or fighting off infection.[186]

Opt Out

Information on the poisonous nature and questionable efficacy of vaccines is available, just not widely available. Vaccines are approved as safe based on flawed studies where the control group is not given a placebo so spikes of adverse reactions in both groups are similar.[187] The National Vaccine Information Center on the web provides an advocacy portal to information on vaccine research. Though not disclosed by doctors, anyone can opt out of vaccination using a waiver for religious reasons or personal conviction. You always have a choice when it comes to health. Under the Precautionary Principle, you can refuse anything that may potentially cause harm.

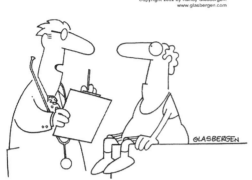

Copyright 2002 by Randy Glasbergen.
www.glasbergen.com

GLASBERGEN

"We can't find anything wrong with you, so we're going to treat you for Symptom Deficit Disorder."

The alternative is to require a medical professional to sign a document ensuring safety and efficacy for vaccines. Ask your healthcare providers to stand behind the products they recommend. Why allow unknown risks to your child's health and well-being without real, longterm safety studies? (See Physician Warranty of Vaccine Safety in Appendix IV).

Chapter Six

THE AGE OF AUTISM

Welcome to the Age of Autism where everyone knows someone living on the autism spectrum. Autism spectrum disorder (ASD) labels those who have difficulties in communication, and social and behavioral skills. Known to be more common among boys than girls,[188] this condition seemed to baffle the medical community for years. As with other conditions, medical research identifies the symptoms but fails to identify a cause.

Parents of vaccine damaged children were the first to notice a clear cause and effect relationship between vaccination and ASD which usually occurred between a visit to the doctor for shots and the sudden breakdown and withdrawal of their child. Many pointed to the toxins in vaccines (mercury and aluminum) identified on the package insert, as a possible cause of autism. While the CDC rejects any link between autism and heavy metals in vaccines, there is published data to back up parents' suspicions that thimerosal in vaccines destroys glutathione, a potent antioxidant necessary for heavy metal detoxification[189] [190] [191] Without glutathione, toxins accumulate and circulate in the body and cross the blood-brain barrier. Glutamic acid in vaccines is another substance also known to destroy glutathione.

Replenishing glutathione may be one key to reversing autism. Glutathione is produced by the body and contains sulfur groups that act like sticky tape that stick to free radicals and heavy metals for removal. Glutathione detoxifies the liver, kidneys, lungs, intestinal epithelia, and other organs. Glutathione is also necessary for lymphocytes, T-cell activation, and is a neurohormone due to its presence in the brain. The body's cells naturally produce glutathione, but the major site of synthesis is in the liver.[192]

There are multiple factors that cause a depletion of glutathione: a poor diet, exposure to heavy metals, environmental toxins, acetaminophen (Tylenol®), household chemicals, stress, trauma, infections, and electromagnetic radiation from cell phone towers, etc., all of which cause the liver to become overburdened as an organ of detoxification. Tylenol®, found in over 600 over-the-counter and prescription meds, is known to cause liver failure and risk of death, especially if taken with alcohol.[193] However, Tylenol also increases the risk of asthma, which seems share parallel aspects of autism and inflammatory disorders.[194] A recent study showed young children who take Tylenol only once a year raise their risk for asthma by seventy percent, while those receiving Tylenol once a month or more were 540 percent more likely to develop asthma.[195] More alarming, acetaminophen use after measles-mumps-rubella vaccination was significantly associated with autistic disorder in children 5 years of age or less.[196] A 2013 study further links Tylenol use during pregnancy to autism.[197]

Glutathione deficiency leads to cell disintegration and is therefore found in all chronic conditions, including autism. Children with autism have lower blood levels of methionine, cysteine, homocysteine and glutathione compared to typical children.[198] Whether toxic exposures come in the form of 1,000 pounds of industrial mercury emissions annually or 25 mcg of mercury in each vaccine, along with added aluminum, there is a clear and significant link between heavy metals in the blood and the condition known as autism.

Kids become poisoned when their bodies can no longer detoxify heavy metals and continue to be exposed. A 2005 US survey using CDC numbers showed the average rate of autism in vaccinated children as one in 166.[199] However, these numbers were based on data collected in 2002. Correcting CDC's numbers for an annual estimated increase of thirteen percent, the autism rate had jumped to one in 78 in 2009.[200] In 2012, the autism rate climbed to one in 67 kids (one in 54 boys). Extrapolating out, autism is expected to rise to a rate of one in eighteen by 2016 and one in nine by 2022.[201]

The symptoms of autism look different in every child, affecting digestive, psychological, and neurologic systems, with symptoms like social withdrawal, reduced eye contact, loss of speech, repetitive behaviors (head banging), seizures, aggression, and no affect (expression). These are the same symptoms identified in children with mercury poisoning. Not surprisingly, the aluminum adjuvants now added to vaccines appear to contribute to the rising prevalence of autism.[202]

Autism is a clear visual of a compromised immune system. In a world where nutrition is lacking, children are fed empty calories, and where human umbilical cord blood is measured to contain over 400 chemicals simply from growing in a human body, vaccination is an added insult to an already compromised immune system. Vaccines are often the last straw that brings on the conditions of asthma, hay fever, neurodermatitis, diabetes, sleep disorders, migraine, bedwetting, hyperactivity, epilepsy, seizures, autoimmune disorders, Celiac's, GERD, gluten sensitivity, thyroid disease, dyslexia, anxiety, sensory processing disorder, depression, and concentration problems.[203]

Dr. Natasha Campbell-McBride, MD, author of "Gut and Psychology Syndrome" writes, "It is the state of the child's immune system that appears to be the decisive factor, not the vaccines." In her own practice she sees children who have not been vaccinated yet exhibit the same conditions; asthma, eczema, ADHD, and autism. However, she believes vaccines may well be the trigger that starts the disorder of autism in immune-compromised children.[204]

An alarming trend is unfolding when comparing the number of vaccines given before age five and the rise in the diagnosis of autism. In 1983 only ten vaccines were given and the autism rate was one in ten thousand. In 2008, the vaccine schedule was increased to 36 vaccines and the autism rate was one in 150. Today, over forty-nine doses of fourteen vaccines are given before kindergarten, 26 doses in the first year.

In England, Gastroenterologist, Dr. Andrew Wakefield, published a study in 1998 presenting clinical evidence for a link between the thimerosal-laden MMR vaccine, intestinal bowel dysfunction, and regressive autism. Earlier in 1961, a German pediatrician and medical theorist named Hans Asperger had made a similar link between mercury poisoning and its associated symptoms. However, Wakefield had gone farther in showing that fragments of the measles viral vaccine were found in the gut of kids with "Leaky Gut."[205]

In the February 2002 *Journal Molecular Pathology*, Dr Wakefield reiterated a link between the measles virus and bowel disease in children with developmental disorders. He concluded that the measles virus may act as a trigger, leading to problems with the immune system. Wakefield was subsequently discredited by the British Medical Authority in 2010 for publicizing his results and lost his license to practice medicine in England. He continues his research in the United States and has the support of a growing number of families living with autism.

In 2012, Dr. Wakefield presented information to the public showing that that the risk for autism had increased to one in 32 children.[206] For all the criticism of Dr. Wakefield's unpopular findings, no single study of health and safety outcomes of vaccinated people versus unvaccinated has yet been conducted to disprove him, either by a government agency or university. In the last fifty years, the schedule of vaccinations for children has only increased. However, Dr. Wakefield has been vindicated based on several recent rulings in Italian and American courts that have awarded compensation to victims of MMR vaccine brain injuries that resulted in autism associated with leaky gut.[207 208 209 210] These landmark decisions have gone mostly unreported except by independent news outlets.

Clinical evidence from independent sources seems to back up Wakefield's conclusions. A 2003 study showed autistic children to have elevated levels of measles antibodies in their bodies.[211] Epidemiological studies conducted by David and Mark Geier using VAERS data from the late '80s through the mid '90s showed a statistically significant link between increasing doses of thimerosal and increasing rates of autism, speech disorders, mental retardation, infantile spasms, and thinking abnormalities in children in the United States.[212 213 214] They also showed a correlation between the number of measles-containing vaccines and autism.[215]

Physical disease results from the interaction between our internal environment and an increasingly toxic external environment. One cannot simply trick the body into immunity using a viral-based chemical soup. The best way to develop a strong immune system is through natural exposure to infectious illness while allowing the body to respond naturally, using all immune pathways to evolve and grow toward homeostasis, as Nature does.

The Gut-Brain Connection

The body is built to be a yin-yang masterpiece, separated in two halves yet connected in such as way that each individual half can partially control the entire body. Similarly, the Mayan Cross describes the body's wholeness as two hemispheres – the right reflecting the material and the left reflecting the spiritual – that merge in a central core of the Self. The body does not need two of every organ to run smoothly, even if we think it might be better to have two brains instead of one.

Wait a few years and things inevitably change. As it turns out, the body really does have two brains – the brain of your head and the brain of your gut, and they are connected to each other. These two brains originate from the same clump of tissue in the embryo called the neural crest. During fetal development, one section becomes the central nervous system and the other migrates to become the enteric nervous system, (ENS), which lies within the folds and lining of esophagus, stomach, small intestine and colon – the gastrointestinal system. The two nervous systems connect via a cable called the vagus nerve – the longest of all the cranial nerves.[216] With the discovery of this gut-brain connection, the study of neurogastroenterology had to be born, which has pushed science to admit that the gut, like the brain, has a mind of its own.

Like the cerebral brain, the gut brain is a network of neurotransmitters, proteins (neuropeptieds) and contains the same number of neurons found in the brain – one hundred million of them – which transfer messages in the same way the higher brain does, so it can learn, act, and remember independently. Gut function actually mirrors brain function, producing a plentiful amount of the neurotransmitters – dopamine, glutamate, norepinephrine, nitric oxide, and serotonin. In fact we now know that ninety-five percent of the body's serotonin is found in the gut, along with the same hormones, natural pain killers, and endorphins. Two brains may be better than one when it comes to pleasure, however, if one brain gets upset, the other one does too.[217]

The vagus nerve controls the rate of messages firing back and forth from brain to brain, and explains why we act and feel the way we do. It explains why a frightening situation will release stress hormones in the gut to give the feeling of "butterflies," while neurons released in the esophagus cause people to "choke" with emotion.[218]

The ENS is the body's second nervous system and acts completely independently from the central nervous system, as seen in stroke victims who can no longer control swallowing. If food is bypassed directly to the stomach, digestion and absorption can take place, even if the person is "brain-dead."

In cases of great stress, the higher brain protects the gut brain by sending signals to mast cells to secrete histamine, prostaglandin, and other agents that help produce inflammation. By inflaming the gut, the brain prepares the gut for surveillance duty so that if the gut lining ends up suffering a leak, the gut is ready to make repairs.

When the body is exposed to a substance, both brains are affected. This explains why people who take antidepressants experience GI problems such as diarrhea, constipation, nausea, and fluctuations in appetite. These drugs prevent the uptake of serotonin to GI cells to make it more available to the brain of a depressed person. However, when there is a reduction in serotonin to calm the gut for a bowel movement (peristalsis), then GI symptoms of cramping, diarrhea, and constipation result. With too much serotonin in the gut, Irritable Bowel Syndrome results.[219]One study showed that a drug preventing the release of serotonin in the gut counteracted osteoporosis, suggesting that, to a degree, the gut regulates bone mass.[220]

As one might expect, morphine and heroin attach to the gut's opiate receptors just like they attach to the brain's opiate receptors, with the added effect of constipation. Both brains can become addicted.[221] This explains why opiates, like laudanum, given as suppositories, travel directly to the source, increasing efficiency.

The same thing happens when a food source becomes an allergen. Mast cells in the gut can become sensitized to antigens in the food. The second time the antigen shows up in the gut, the mast cells call up a program, releasing chemical modulators that try to eliminate the threat. The allergic person experiences diarrhea and cramps.

The gut-brain connection supports the notion that our body coordinates innate intelligence, and counterintelligence, in order to maintain balance. The body knows intrinsically how to react under any threat. And as science catches up to the wisdom of the body, it has the opportunity for developing microbial treatments for brain conditions.

Such strategies would recognize that healthy gut bacteria regulate normal brain development as well as behavior. When you are happy it is because your levels of brain serotonin (happy hormones) are being directed by the amount and type of bacteria in your gut. One study showed that the sooner in life good bacteria are established in the gut, the more likely happiness is maintained throughout adulthood without the need for antidepressants, which work by targeting this hormone.[222]

Science is slowly recognizing that autism reflects a neurological assault on the gut-brain microbial axis via a toxic exposure to an already compromised immune system. In short, toxic bacterial byproducts are getting through to the brain, bypassing both the intestinal barrier and the blood-brain barrier. Autism studies demonstrate that the vagal nerve is affected, which not only means beat-to-beat regulation is impaired, but there is also brain stem malfunction. This results in a decrease in the brain's state of arousal that manifests in the lack of affect and facial expression.[223] More information on the mechanism of this reaction can be found in Dr. Wakefield's books *Callous Disregard: Autism and Vaccines, The Truth Behind A Tragedy,* and *Waging War on the Autistic Child: The Arizona 5 And The Legacy of Baron von Munchausen.*

Chapter Seven

INDUSTRIAL FOOD, INDUSTRIAL HEALTH

Despite living in the age of prosperity, Americans are sicker than ever before. Not only are we less healthy than our counterparts in other developed countries,[224] but the baby boom generation is now in worse shape than their parents.[225] And teens, for the first time in history are making their parents look good.[226]

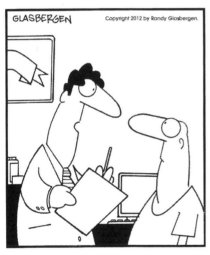

"The good news is, you have the heart of a teenager. The bad news is, most teenagers these days have the heart of an old man."

Despite the most expensive health care system in the world, data from the World Health Organization and the Organization for Economic Cooperation and Development shows that Americans rank last out of seventeen nations when it comes to health.[227] Not only do more Americans die from injuries, homicides, and alcohol and other drugs, but we can take credit for the highest rates of heart disease, lung disease, obesity, and diabetes.[228] American deaths disproportionately affect the young, as seen by the highest rankings for infant mortality rate, pregnancy complications, and death before age five. The research uncovered no single cause accounting for the totality of America's ill health, yet argued, as research always does, that more research is needed.

The economics of 'more research is needed' means billions of research dollars continue to roll through the academic doors, even if it also means that serious scholarly thinking has left the room. Anyone using three percent of his brain can clearly deduce that Americans are overfed and undernourished because the food of the 21st century lacks minerals and nutrients. The chemical soup in which we live exposes us to more toxins on a daily basis than our ancestors were exposed during a lifetime. Bombarded by toxins in our air, water, and food, the body is further depleted of essential minerals, and compensates by increasing fat stores for protection of its organs.

Without the right complement of minerals and microbes, the body lacks the tools necessary to repair and rebuild its cells on a minute-by-minute basis. Minerals are the catalysts of vitamins and co-nutrients of enzymes in the body for most biological reactions. The most important minerals needed by the body include: iron, copper, zinc, chromium, phosphorus, sulfur, magnesium, manganese, potassium, iodine, selenium, and molybdenum, that function to:

- help maintain acid-base balance, to keep the body pH neutral.
- become part of tissue structure, such as in bone and teeth.
- help regulate body processes, such as in enzyme systems.
- function in nerve impulse transmission and muscle contraction.
- help release energy from food.

"You can trace every sickness, every disease, and every ailment to a mineral deficiency."

~Linus Pauling, nobel laureate in chemistry

Loss of Minerals

Mineral deficiencies should be a main concern for human health. A single mineral deficiency can create an imbalance which leads to disease. There are many causes for the loss of minerals, including:

1) Mineral-deficient soils resulting from industrial agricultural strip-mining practices, and more recently by GMO pesticides and herbicides.

2) Dietary choices (processed foods devoid of minerals) and inorganic forms of mineral supplements that are not absorbed or bioavailable to the body. For instance, the milling of wheat destroys forty percent of the chromium, eight percent of the cobalt, sixty-eight percent of the copper, seventy-eight percent of the zinc, and forty-eight percent of the molybdenum. And white bread turns to glucose as quickly as white sugar.[229]

3) Overuse of prescription drugs (Tylenol®, Advil®, Motrin®, aspirin, etc.,) all inhibit mineral absorption across the intestine wall. The body further depletes its mineral reserves in metabolizing and detoxifying the body of laxatives, diuretics, chemotherapy, and NSAIDs.

4) Reduced function of elimination organs to prevent uptake of minerals, especially due to a buildup of mucoid plaque along the lining of the colon wall.

5) Competition of minerals in the body. Any excess of one mineral may cause a deficiency of another, as in the case of iron, copper, and zinc. A lack of copper causes secondary iron deficiency. Zinc and copper compete for absorption from the intestine into the blood. An excess of zinc reduces copper. Copper deficiency is a risk factor for osteoporosis, rheumatoid arthritis and cardiovascular disease, as well as high rates of colds and flu, reproductive issues, and fatigue.

One of the first studies recognizing the incontrovertible importance of minerals was published in JAMA in 1996, showing powerful antioxidant properties and anti-tumorigenic effects of selenium (200 mcg organic selenium) when taken at levels higher than normal nutritional needs. In this case-controlled study of 1,312 subjects, there were impressive reductions of sixty-three percent for prostate cancer, fifty-eight percent for colon-rectal cancers, and forty-six for lung cancer.

The study was terminated early so that everyone could begin to benefit from selenium.[230]

Simply put, when minerals go down, disease goes up. Disease prevalence in both plants and humans goes back to the soil. Soil pH determines the soil mineral content and whether plants thrive or fail. If the soil is too acid, minerals are dissolved too quickly and carried away as water drains. If soil is too alkaline, not enough minerals dissolve and they become bound up. The healthiest soil, where minerals are available for plant uptake is found at a pH of 6.7 (neutral).

In humans, too, all physiologic processes are pH sensitive. Research is clear that "acidification is a common finding in fluids associated with inflammation throughout the body."[231, 232, 233] Most people today have created acidic inner terrains which sets up a chain reaction toward inflammation of the pancreas (diabetes), the brain (neurologic conditions), the heart (heart disease), and every other system. Each bodily fluid has an optimal pH, so when bodily tissues become too acidic (pH too low), metabolism speeds up, and likewise, when the body becomes too alkaline (pH too high), metabolism slows down.

Mineral deficient plants now contain toxic residues that can no longer simply be washed off foods because they are integrated within the genome of ninety percent of foods in the western diet as GMOs. A 2013 study published in the *Journal Entropy* showed Roundup Ready, a glyphosate-based, GMO herbicide, interrupts the metabolic pathway of our bacteria in the same way it does of the plants, causing two key problems – nutritional deficiencies and systemic toxicity[234] GMO food crops of concern include sugar beets, corn, canola (rape seed), alfalfa, cottonseed, soybeans, papaya, milk, Aspartame®, and more recently, wheat. Aspartame® and glyphosate are now banned in most countries around the world. Here's why:

Aspartame

Aspartame® – Nutra Sweet®, Equal®, Splenda® – is an artificial sweetener 200 times sweeter than sugar, used in the United States since the early 1980s. It is added to thousands of food products and diet soda, and most recently to processed milk as a "low-calorie" sweetener. Made from the waste products of genetically modified E. coli bacteria, it is known to cause brain tumors in rats and is likely to be a cause of spasms, numbness, cramps, headaches, tinnitus, joint pain, depression, anxiety attacks, and blurred vision in humans. Methanol is released from Aspartame® within hours of ingestion, is carried in the blood, into the brain and bone marrow and converted into formaldehyde where it damages sensitive myelin tissue (nerves) and proteins including DNA.[235] It is a cumulative poison, meaning it accumulates without being efficiently excreted. Multiple Sclerosis may be misdiagnosed as Aspartame poisoning since many of those who come off diet sodas often experience a complete reversal of symptoms.

"Nothing else does in your brain quite like diet cola. This is because there is a deadly combination of aspartame and caffeine, and together they create a very unique blend of excitotoxin that kills off brain cells."

~Dr. Christiane Northrup, Hungry for Change Film

Glyphosate

Glyphosate is pervasive in the processed food supply. Its action in the body effectively destroys our populations of beneficial gut bacteria. The resulting toxins create Leaky Gut and inflammation, which lead to gastrointestinal disorders (IBD, colitis), mood swings, Alzheimer's, Parkinson's, infertility, allergies (e.g., wheat), autism, heart disease, diabetes, and all types of cancer.[236] It is no coincidence that gut disorders seemed to increase worldwide when the application of Roundup herbicide became popular in the mid-1990s.

The claims that GMO corn is no different from non-GMO corn have been proven false in a 2012 Corn Comparison Report that revealed that glyphosate draws out the nutrients from living foods, leaving corn nutritionally dead. Results showed non-GMO corn to have seven times more manganese, 56 times more magnesium, and 437 times more calcium than GMO corn. These are the same deficiencies identified in people diagnosed with disorders from osteoporosis to cancer. GMO corn also has high levels of formaldehyde that animals can smell, the reason why they refuse to eat it.[237] For all the industry marketing that touts the benefits and safety of GMO foods, our bodies do not suffer from a deficiency of toxic heavy metals and chemicals and neither does Nature. In losing a conscious connection to the soil and our food, we all end up suffering the consequences.

Human Costs of Industrial Life

Currently, more than 133 million Americans, about fifty percent of the population, have at least one chronic condition, and twenty-six percent have multiple chronic conditions. Chronic disease is the leading cause of death and responsible for seventy percent of all death and disability in the United States.[238]

Research from the Mayo Clinic shows that seventy percent of Americans take at least one prescription drug, more than fifty percent take at least two prescriptions, and twenty percent take five or more prescription medications, the most commonly prescribed being antibiotics, antidepressants, and painkiller opioids.[239] The author of the study, Dr. St. Sauver reported the obvious findings without blinking: "As you get older you tend to get more prescriptions, and women tend to get more prescriptions than men." The NIH on Aging and the Mayo Clinic funded the study to tell us something we already knew without suggesting a cause or a solution. Equally impressive to our drug-induced stupor is the economic burden related to treatment costs for chronic disease, estimated at $1.7 trillion annually, about three-quarters of total health care dollars spent, or about twenty percent of the nation's Gross Domestic Product (GDP).[240]

The endless drug pipeline, with its corresponding pipeline of bio-tech stocks, reflects bio- business treating the conditions of industrial life even as hundreds of FDA-approved drugs are recalled every year for toxicity. Often new drugs block naturally occurring proteins of cell metabolism, and then are later made obsolete due to the discovery that those protein are in the body for a reason, as in the case of Alzheimer's.[241] Or it is found that long-term use of antidepressants (tricyclic, MAOI, SSRI) is associated with a two-fold greater risk of diabetes.[242]

A worrisome trend is seen by the increase in childhood obesity, which has tripled in the United States over the past twenty years, resulting in the quadrupling of childhood chronic diseases in the past four decades. Due to this trend, the next generation of Americans is at a greater risk for developing chronic disease.

Welcome to the modern American lifestyle where the more you see the doctor, the more you see the doctor, and where the cost to do so is projected to reach $4.3 trillion by 2016. While the United States rivals the rest of the world in providing the best trauma care through its emergency rooms, the rest of the medical system is failing us. When a July 26, 2000, JAMA article reported that Western medicine is the third leading cause of death in the United States it appeared to be a conservative estimate as only a fraction of iatrogenic (medically-caused) deaths are ever reported.

"I went to the doctor with a problem. I came out with a disease."

~Groucho Marx

How do we explain the growing numbers who appear healthy, but suffer from food intolerances and autoimmune disease? What about the increases in death rates from all forms of cancer? Why does the body insist on attacking itself?

The broad answer is that we have lost our connection to Nature. The rise in obesity, the accumulation of fat on the body, is a way the body naturally protects itself against an onslaught of heavy metals and chemicals by keeping them out of the blood. Obesity also reflects an imbalance of our microbes and/or the loss of beneficial microbes. All chronic disease is a reflection of the lost integrity of the body's immune system. But de-naturing from our planet is only part of the problem. The other part is our agreement with how medical science classifies diseases based on a list of symptoms and then suppresses those symptoms with chemical-based drugs without addressing the cause. While each condition appears to be different, the truth is that they all represent a continuum of symptoms from a cascade of organ system failures that result from one main cause – a compromised immune system from an imbalance in intestinal gut flora.[243]

"Treat the cause not the effect."

~Dr. Edward Bach, creator of flower essences

Food Intolerances on Rise

New diseases appear to be nothing more than new expressions of the same root causes. Dis-ease not only reflects too much food, or the wrong foods, but not enough of the right foods. Nutritional deficiencies in food are a modern day concern, just as they were in the past. A lack of nutrients in our food weakens our immune systems and shows up as symptoms.

For instance, a vitamin D deficiency results in Rickets but can also lead to autoimmune conditions like Type 1 diabetes,[244] and rheumatoid arthritis.[245] A lack of iodine is known to result in goiter, an enlargement of the thyroid, but it is also primarily responsible for autoimmune thyroid disease, fibrocystic disease, and breast and prostate cancer.[246] Vitamin A deficiency is known to cause visual impairment and night blindness, but it also leads to the body's inability to fight infections. Dr. Carey Reams, from his ionization research, showed that leukemia is due in large part to a lack of vitamin A, which means poor absorption in the gut.

With food intolerances on the rise over the past fifty years due to the industrial matrix in which we live, new diseases are constantly being named and classified. However, if the goal is to heal the body and reverse disease, then it is not the classification by itself that is important but the cause.

In his book, *The Ultimate Healing System*, Donald Lepore, ND, says each allergic substance is really a response by the body to deficiencies of specific vitamins, minerals, fatty acids, carbohydrates, and amino acids. Without these vital nutrients, complete absorption of the food does not occur.

A milk "allergy" or lactose intolerance reflects a mineral deficiency due to deficient dairy. Labeling someone as "lactase deficient" wrongly blames the victim for a problem that originates with processed milk which removes most minerals, enzymes and nutrients. The body comes with only a limited supply of enzymes and, therefore, depends on food to supply its own for complete digestion. Pasteurization eliminates all inherent enzymes, including the phosphatase enzyme necessary for the absorption of calcium, the main reason to drink milk. The resulting symptoms (gas, bloating, cramping, diarrhea, constipation, vomiting, and weak bones) are the body's innate intelligence responding when faced with a substance that is deficient and thereby inherently toxic.

For people who are seemingly "allergic" to everything, Lepore says sodium and potassium levels have become depleted. This can result from sweating during summer activities and from eating non-nutritious foods. Eating more greens or raw celery, high in organic sodium, as well as raw carrots and bananas, which are high in potassium, can help to correct the problem. Both minerals are critical for all cells to maintain balance.

A significant portion of the population today not only reacts to dairy, but also to gluten. Studies are showing that these reactions cause the immune system to destroy brain and nervous tissue in "neurological autoimmunity" as seen by positive tissue antibodies in Alzheimer's, Parkinson's, autism, childhood development disorders.[247] Because wheat has been altered to create a hardier, "new and improved" pest resistant grain, it can no longer be digested, and thereby builds resistance in the body. This causes mutagenic changes at the site of incorporation in the small intestine, which first shows itself as Irritable Bowel Syndrome. Antibodies pass through the blood-brain barrier to affect the brain. Jeffrey Smith, director of the Institute of Responsible Technology suggests a link between GMOs in the food supply and gluten-related disorders.[248] Choosing not to eat wheat at all is becoming a necessity to health. (See more in Appendix II, Go Gluten-free).

In their book *Dangerous Grains*, Braly and Hoggan write that chromium deficiency is a major contributor to the rise of both Celiac's disease (gluten intolerance) and diabetes mellitus, each classified as autoimmune. Often these conditions are seen together and reflect a deficiency of chromium glucose tolerance factor (GTF). Chromium is essential to maintaining stable blood sugar levels and also improves insulin efficiency for glucose metabolism. It helps make the body's own insulin go further. A similar autoimmune reaction is seen in diabetes mellitus type 2, previously tied solely to poor diet and inactivity.[249]When up to of ninety percent of Americans consume less than the minimal fifty micrograms of chromium a day, it follows that Celiacs eating a typical western diet, high in refined flour and sugar, would be profoundly chromium deficient. Chromium deficiency, as seen in diabetes mellitus types 1 and 2, is also seen in hyperglycemia hyperinsulinism, gestational diabetes (diabetes of pregnancy), and corticosteroid-induced diabetes.[250] While supplementation with chromium alone may not completely reverse diabetes mellitus, many studies have shown that chromium polynicotinate or chromium picolinate are forms that improve insulin function and can lead to improved glucose tolerance.[251] However, whole-food GTF chromium supplementation is arguably the most beneficial because it comes from food.[252]

Autoimmune Disease on the Rise

Food intolerances reflect a lack of nutrients in a weakened immune system. With the addition of toxins that mimic the body's own cells, the body is misguided into attacking itself, resulting in autoimmunity. Most people wouldn't be able to name a single autoimmune disease if asked. But there are at least 100 such conditions, all of which have their root in Leaky Gut. Here are a few:[253] [254] [255]

Asthma
Autism
Ataxia
Atopic Dermatitis
Autism Spectrum Disorders
Bipolar Disorder
Autoimmune Thyroiditis
Casein Intolerance
Celiac's Disease
Chronic Fatigue Syndrome
Cirrhosis: Liver
Conjunctival tumor
Dermatitis
Depression
Diabetes Mellitus Type 1
Down's Syndrome
Eosinophilic esophagitis
Eczema
Food Allergies
Giardiasis
Graves Disease
Huntington's Disease
Hyperthyroidism
Infertility

Inflammatory Bowel Disease
Kidney Cancer
Liver Disease
Lymphoma
Malnutition
Multiple Sclerosis
Psoriasis
Recurrent Miscarriage
Rheumatoid arthritis
Reiter's Syndrome
Meniere's Disease
Migraine Disorders
Peripheral Neuropathies
Pituitary Diseases
Polyarthritis
Psychiatric Disorders
Psoriasis
Parkinson's
Schizophrenia
Sjogren's Syndrome
Systemic Lupus erythematosa
Thyroid disease
Ulcerative colitis

Chapter Eight

NATURAL MEDICINE

In the fifth century Hippocrates said, "The natural healing force within each of us is the greatest force in getting well." Fifteen centuries later, Linus Pauling moved this idea forward with ortho-molecular medicine – "the treatment of disease by the provision of the optimum molecular environment, especially the optimum concentrations of substances normally present in the human body." Physician and agronomist, Dr. Carey Reams, later showed the cause of every disease relates to mineral deficiencies and that every disease is reversible by replenishing the body with the appropriate minerals.

The five thousand year-old philosophies of ayruvedic medicine and traditional Chinese Medicine, and the more recent disciplines of naturopathy and homeopathy, each recognize, respect, and honor the human connection to Nature. They understand the body to be self-sustaining under natural conditions, and that uncovering and addressing toxicities and nutritional deficiencies is a first step in addressing core imbalances to restore full health. They look for windows of opportunity to prevent disease before it takes hold. As we make our way in life, disease becomes a choice. We can prevent it now or react to it later. We have the "cure" because we know the cause. The biggest part of the problem has been sheer ignorance. But that is curable too.

"All symptoms of so-called diseases have but one cause. All diseases are one. Unity in all things is nature's plan. The human body is a holistic entity and must be treated as such."

~Robert J. Thiel, Ph.D, N.D.

One Cause of Disease

The Law of Unity of Disease says there is only one cause of disease called toxemia, a condition in which a toxin – from junk food, products of metabolism, chemical, heavy metal, a compacted colon, etc., – moves through the blood then deeper into the body. This Train of Disease shows how all disease conditions are really one disease. If we could catch the Train of Disease on a virtual tour through the body we would see that disease in the blood is seen as inflammation. From the blood, the toxin spreads to all cells and the weaker tissues. Symptoms of gastr*itis* or cyst*itis* or arthr*itis* are the body's expression of imbalance-by-location in attempts to eliminate the toxin from the blood. Simply put, acute inflammation is the body's natural defense to a foreign invader. However, once the body is chronically exposed to toxins or wrong foods, chronic inflammation and physical injury result.

"Without inflammation, cholesterol would move freely throughout the body as nature intended. It is inflammation that causes cholesterol to become trapped."[255]

~Dwight Lundell, M.D.

The injury and inflammation of coronary artery disease so common in the 21st century is caused by a low fat diet which has been recommended for years by mainstream medicine. The main dietary culprits are processed and refined sugar, flour, and the overuse of vegetable oils (corn, canola, soy, and sunflower). The label 'atherosclerosis' simply reflects the body attempt to heal itself from injury.[257] The buildup of cholesterol arrives to the scene in the same fashion fire trucks arrive to the scene of a fire; after the fire has already started.

Under natural conditions, the body's intelligence works to limit damage to organs by keeping symptoms at the surface. The skin is the first area in which symptoms appear. Therefore, to treat the skin, the inner problems need to be addressed. The founder of Homeopathy Samuel Hahnemann believed that suppression of rashes or psoriasis with steroidal creams only drives the problem deeper to become more serious diseases.[258] In fact, most products that come into contact with the skin go directly to the bloodstream without the benefit of being filtered through the digestive tract. So it makes sense to only put on the skin what Nature provides (clean water, coconut, almond, jojoba oils, some essential oils, certain clays, egg whites, herbal salves, etc.).

This train-of-thought describes disease as a series of symptoms produced by the body as it attempts to rid the toxins through the mucous membranes in what appears to be healing efforts. Once the body throws off the toxemia, all diseases are reversed. Removal of a toxin through the mucous membranes of the nose is called a cold.

"You can't keep one disease and heal two others. When the body heals, it heals everything."

~Charlotte Gerson, The Gerson Institute

Over two thousand years ago, when Hippocrates devised the Law of Cure, he said, "Every acute disease is the result of a cleansing and healing effort by Nature." Common colds, infections, fevers, and pneumonias are Nature's effort to eliminate toxins from its ecosystem. An acute disease is nothing more than a "healing reaction" since such reactions do not develop under normal, healthy conditions. For chronic conditions where toxins are found at deeper levels, we can help Nature along using tools that jump-start the healing process. Removal of toxins from the colon is assisted using a colonic. The removal of toxins from the liver is called an enema.

Stepping back to look at the big picture, we see how beliefs on healing have been driven by two different languages. Whereas Western medicine drives the toxin deeper with drugs based on fear of the germ, natural medicine strives to rid the body of toxins through trusting the body's innate intelligence. Nature's pathways include:

1) raising body temperature to burn out foreign invaders; 2) nourishing the body with healing foods to boost the immune system; 3) eliminating toxins via the liver, lungs, kidneys, colon, and skin; 4) avoiding future toxins, and 5) rest.

In natural medicine, the blood is viewed as a ground-floor window to the effects of a person's lifestyle and habits. If the blood is pure, no pathogens – viruses, parasites, yeast, bad bacteria – will survive, and no disease is possible. However, if the blood is not pure, then the cause of our dis-ease has everything to do with our choices – what we eat, breathe, drink, inject, think, feel, and do.

Planet Earth provides for all the body's needs in order to live in full health, assuming we get what we need from the packages Nature provides. Contrary to medical theory, the liver, pancreas, saliva, and small intestine do not create all the enzymes our bodies need. Cultural differences reveal wide variations in the enzymes the body is able to manufacture. The body expects most of its enzymes to come with the food. Yet processing, sterilization, irradiation, genetic engineering, and heating all destroy the digestive enzymes found in fresh, whole, live foods. Without food enzymes, our bodies go above and beyond the call of duty until our enzymes are gone. Partially digested food makes its way into the blood where the body's counter-intelligence forces begin the attack in a friendly fire scenario as they are designed to do.

Nature provides for all of our body's needs in the form of healthy, living, enzyme-rich, nutrient-dense, foods from a varied diet of organic foods. Only with real food can our bodies make the repairs to maintain health. Health is the body in its natural state. True health is body, mind, and spirit living in harmony with Nature's elements – fire, earth, water, and air – broken down as carbon, nitrogen, oxygen, and hydrogen. Real food is comprised of these elements in the form of vitamins, minerals, amino acids, fatty acids, carbohydrates, and enzymes. If nutrients are not provided or replenished, the body compensates, one organ system taking from another in order to balance itself. A chain reaction of organ system failures occurs resulting in disharmony for the whole. The body responds naturally with what it is given or not given.

"The treatments themselves do not 'cure' the condition, they simply restore the body's self-healing ability."

~Leon Chaitow, N.D. D.O. "
Alternative Medicine the Definitive Guide"

Naturopathy

Naturopathy is the science, art, and philosophy of Nature. Naturopaths focus on the prevention of disease using a mix of whole foods, diet and nutrition, herbs, cleansing tools, the sun, air, water, rest, as well as homeopathics and Bach Flower remedies. Full health can be restored without suppressing the vital life force with inorganic substances, drugs, synthetic chemicals, surgery, toxins, serums, inoculations, or radiation. Naturopaths teach about the laws of Nature and natural living so that each individual understands personal responsibility for making choices for health, in recognition that the body heals itself on multiple levels. Natural medicine teaches us to honor and embrace health as our natural birthright so there is no need to fear disease.

Homeopathy

Homeopathy stimulates a person's immune system to heal under Samuel Hahnemann's Law of Similars, where "like is cured by like." There are about 6,000 homeopathic remedies on the market today, each specific to a substance (plant, mineral, toxin, pathogen, pesticide) that reflects a profile of symptoms. The effect of a remedy mirrors the symptom of the disease to target the invader. Remedies are created through a series of dilution and shaken in a process called 'succussion,' which renders the substance 'potentized,' leaving only traces of the original substance in the final solution. The more dilute the solution, the more potent the cure. A common 30C solution is a dilution by a factor of 10^{60}. This energized medicine contains only the essence, which renders it harmless because it heals at the etheric, or energetic, level.

The power of 'potentisation' is seen through one of the largest homeopathic prophylaxis (HP) intervention studies ever undertaken (over 11 million people) conducted against Leptospirosis (Weil's Disease), an infectious disease caused by a spirochete carried by the rat. During an epidemic in three provinces of Cuba in 2007, homeopathic medicine was given to the provinces most affected. "Within a few weeks the number of cases had fallen from thirty-eight to four cases per 100,000 per week, significantly fewer than the historically-based forecast for those weeks of the year." The population without treatment experienced the predicted incidence. The effect of the remedy carried over to the following year (2008) where an 84% reduction in infection was observed in the treated region and "for the first time, incidence did not correlate with the rainy season. In the same period, incidence in the untreated region increased by 22%,"[259] showing how homeopathy both reverses and prevents disease.

Hering's Law

The stunning successes seen when Nature is consulted is explained by the principles of Hering's Law, named after American Homeopath Constantine Hering, M.D. who, in the 1800s, observed that healing happens in a reliable pattern, summarized in three basic laws:

- The first law: healing progresses from the deepest part of the organism - the mental and emotional levels and the vital organs - to the external parts, such as skin and extremities.
- The second law: As healing progresses, symptoms appear and disappear in the reverse of their original order of appearance.
- The third law –healing progresses from the upper to the lower parts of the body.

The healing reaction is known as the "Herxheimer Reaction," or feeling worse before feeling better. It is an immune system reaction to the toxins (endotoxins) that are released when large amounts of pathogens are killed off. Flu-like symptoms can erupt, lasting for a few days before you feel stronger.[260] Healing happens as past illnesses are revealed and unpeeled like layers of an onion. With each reaction, the body gains strength and moves toward full health.

The Energy of Health and Disease

From his work of the 1920s, naturopath Dr. Victor G. Rocine understood the body from a different perspective. He found that health and disease represent different frequencies of vibration.

Rocine found that organs or tissues that lack certain elements altered its electromagnetic field and thus reflected disease. In his work with plants, he found that specific frequencies of certain foods could raise the frequencies of certain tissues in the body to restore them to normal. The vibrations between the food and the body were linked electromagnetically, one vibration indicating a need, and the other indicating the fulfillment of the need. Without the right elements coming from plants (or herbs), each organ becomes unbalanced and cannot play its role in the overall functioning of the body. Rocine understood that minerals in foods are naturally potentized, similar to homeopathic remedies.

What Rocine describes is an attunement between the physical body, the energetic "subtle" body, and the vibrations of many natural remedies. It is the life force of the remedies (homeopathics, flower essences, plants) that cleanse imbalances in the aura (subtle energy field of a person) to correct the physical imbalances that contribute to poor health. This happens because quartz-like crystalline structures in the body – found in cell salts, fatty tissue, lymph, red and white blood cells, and the pineal gland – are amplified by the life force of the remedies. The remedies balance the various organs at the correct frequencies to stimulate the body to discharge the toxin in favor of health.[261]

Like Hahnemann's law of similars, the more correct the mineral balance, the easier it is to attract more of the same. The universal law of attraction, expressed as like attracts like, reflects this energetic concept. Each mineral naturally migrates to be stored in the area in which it is "charged." In this way, calcium is stored in the bones. Sodium is stored in the digestive system. Silicon is stored in the hair, skin, nails, and connective tissue. Magnesium is stored in the muscles, and so on. Understanding these associations, symptoms of skin itching or brittle nails can be targeted with the right frequencies through silicon-containing foods, herbal supplements, homeopathic remedies, essential oils, and other vibrational remedies for self-healing.[262]

Pasteur Recants Germ Theory

Since the advent of antibiotics less than one hundred years ago, it seems we have failed to appreciate what Louis Pasteur, himself, finally understood about the body's immune system. On his deathbed, he fully recanted his Germ Theory. At the end of his life, Pasteur stated, *"It is not the germ that causes disease but the terrain in which the germ is found,"* meaning it is the strength of the immune system and its diversity of good bacteria that determines health or disease. To think that we as a species can kill off the versatility and resilience of the bugs that make up most of the body is an example of not using our whole brain. To this day, Pasteur's rival Bechamp has never been disproved. Bechamp's theory has only been reinforced by further research.

Hygiene Hypothesis

Although the truth about the germ had been conveniently buried under the Germ Theory for a few hundred years, truth always finds a way. In 1989, David Strachan proposed the hygiene hypothesis which suggests what farmers have known for centuries: lack of stimulation of our immune systems by bacteria or viruses early in life can lead to higher rates of allergies and asthma. These diseases were non-existent in the 19th century just as they are in third-world countries today. Without a healthy dose of soil bacteria, we are more likely to develop digestive disease, chronic illnesses, and other disorders of the immune system.[263]

The high rates of appendicitis in industrialized nations is a clear visual of the Hygiene Hypothesis come to life. An inflamed appendix reflects a congested colon from chronic constipation, which must be cleared out naturally with changes in diet and lifestyle. The word appendix comes from the word appendage because western medicine believed the appendix was evolutionarily unnecessary. Whether or not it would become inflamed, it was often removed preventatively as an irrelevant organ. However, like your tonsils and adenoids, the appendix is part of your immune system. It not only secretes white blood cells and antibacterial substances into the colon, it also incubates beneficial bacteria which are released to repopulate the lining of the intestine after the bowel is emptied and before more harmful bacteria can take up residence.[264] No organ in the body is useless even if science has not yet come to understand its purpose.

Exposure to these bugs early in life seems to be a critical factor in the development of healthy immune systems.[265] Later in life, reversals of Crohn's disease, multiple sclerosis, diabetes, and other autoimmune conditions have been achieved by adding probiotics, fermented foods, and supplements to the diet while removing harmful foods. Reversals have also been seen using helminthic therapy (i.e., parasitic worms).[266] Introducing the eggs of whipworms into the body helps to redirect a mis-firing immune system to normalcy. Instead of attacking itself, the body attacks what it is supposed to attack.[267]

Deficient Tests

Blood is the window to the body's health. However, allopathic medicine's main diagnostic tool of the blood test has its limits and is not always sensitive enough to tell the whole story. If not providing clues to the cause of disease, the blood test only serves to maintain disease.

For instance, various B vitamin deficiencies can exist while serum levels appear normal.[268] In cases of iron anemia, serum iron levels may appear within range when serum ferritin (iron stores) may be well below normal.[269] Thyroid panels for hormones (T3, T4, TSH) often show false negatives, even when low thyroid function exists since TSH can lag way behind the appearance of low thyroid symptoms.[270] [271]

The blood test is also poor indicator of some essential minerals that reside elsewhere in the body, such as magnesium, which is found primarily in muscles. It is no coincidence that more than eighty percent of the population suffers from magnesium deficiency, the symptoms of which include muscle cramps, bronchial and heart muscle spasms, (i.e., restless leg syndrome), muscle spasms, anxiety, poor memory, confusion, high blood pressure, and potassium deficiency. Magnesium works in concert with calcium and is balanced in the body in a recommended 1:2 ratio with calcium.

The best way to ensure you have enough magnesium in the body is to eat high magnesium foods (spinach, squash, black beans, okra, pumpkin seeds, cashews, almonds, sunflower seeds, raw milk from grass-fed cows) and to supplement transdermally with magnesium chloride, magnesium sulfate (Epsom salt baths), or magnesium citrate, one of the most absorbable forms of magnesium. You'll know you've replenished your magnesium supply when you experience a loose stool; at that point, simply back off on supplementation.[272]

Likewise, in autism evaluations, tests for glutathione levels do not differentiate between active (reduced) and inactive (oxidized) forms. Normal total glutathione level could be misleading since this could be mostly as the oxidized form. "If cysteine is low, then improving the amount of cysteine in the body can help the body make glutathione. But a normal or high cysteine level does not ensure that glutathione levels in the body are accurate." Testing for sulfates is important since low levels of sulfate can lead to toxic accumulation and inflammation. This can be corrected by taking an Epsom salt bath or taking oral sulfates.[273]

Unfortunately, the blood sample Western medicine relies upon is chemically deactivated and altered under a glass slide and is therefore limited in what it can reveal. Basing a diagnosis solely on a blood sample is misleading. Too often, when the answer is not clear the prescription of choice is an antidepressant. When we tunnel our vision to merely track symptoms (acne, low blood pressure, allergies, poor circulation, joint pain, depression, joint pain, muscle weakness, chronic fatigue) which are shared by many organ dysfunctions, we "miss the train" of disease – the underlying cause based in nutrient deficiencies and toxicities. We fail to see the value of our blood as a window to our health. We fail to recognize that the body's elimination pathways are blocked.

Live Blood Analysis

Live blood analysis is the open window that allows for early intervention by showing the opportunity for the prevention and early reversal of disease conditions. This visual tool shows a snapshot of the quality, mobility, and interaction of live blood cells in their natural environment. As a qualitative tool, it shows signs of any bacteria or fungal infection, leaky gut, liver stress, dysbiosis, poor protein digestion, and crystals of uric acid, a sign of inflammation, among other signs. Using dark field microscopy, one drop of blood shows if cells and platelets are misshapen and clumped together, stagnant in blood flow, or if they are fully round and plump, moving without restriction. Live blood cells contain vital life force and give a clear picture of true health. No chemical fixative or eight-year medical degree can do that.

Living blood tells the story of life: a poor diet, excesses of sugar, caffeine, alcohol, changes in pH, and stress. Our blood is not only reflective of our genetics but of our epigenetics. Most all chronic pain lodged in the body derives from chronic inflammatory molecules brought on by how we handle stress. The accumulation of junk in our homes is a metaphor for toxins in our bodies and minds. The answers to the cause of our dis-ease is staring us squarely in the face if we will only open our eyes.

Chapter Nine

THE RE-NATURING PROCESS

French historian Jules Michelet, first coined the term Renaissance around 1855 to describe the rebirth of humanity in the 16th century and its rightful place in the world. He wrote, "You are one of the forces of Nature." Each day is an opportunity for rebirth and rejuvenation. We only need to look to Nature's example of detoxification to see how balance is restored in the body.

One way Nature detoxifies is through electrical storms. Thunder and lightning produce an abundance of negative ions and ozone (O3). As an energized form of oxygen, ozone is Nature's great purifier. It is the free electron of a single O1 oxygen atom from an unstable O3 molecule that has the power to detoxify the most polluted environments because O1 electrons are attracted to positively charged pollutants. During a lightening storm all pollution is completely cleansed. You can smell the clean air. In the same way, ozone converts raw sewage into pure drinking water. The reason we can live on Earth is because the planet is surrounded by ozone.

Ozone is designed by Nature to annihilate toxins whether outside or inside the body. Lack of oxygen in the external environment leads to the loss of aquatic and terrestrial life. Oxygen deficient air means our cells will also be deprived. Symptoms of oxygen starvation (ninety-four percent oxygen or lower) include: memory loss, depression, anxiety, muscle aches, poor digestion and absorption, lowered immunity, and tumors. With enough oxygen, cells naturally generate ozone and hydrogen peroxide (oxidants) to cleanse themselves. The O1 atom combines with anything – viruses, parasites, fungus – without anti-oxidant (enzyme) protection. When cells are one hundred percent oxygenated, the body achieves full energy (chi).

Two-time Nobel Laureate Dr. Otto Warburg proved in 1966 that the prime cause of cancer was the replacement of cellular respiration of oxygen (oxidative phosphorylation) by the fermentation of sugar (glycolysis).[274] Warburg taught that ozone, as a free radical scavenger, destroys diseased cells and foreign invaders that live in anaerobic (no oxygen) conditions. Like iodine and silver, ozone is an anti-fungal, anti-microbial, anti-viral agent. It kills the bad actors without harming the good. As a therapeutic agent, ozone "accelerates brain repair, relieves brain fog, improves circulation, purifies the skin, boosts immune function, stimulates enzyme activity, and stimulates killer cell activity, as it detoxifies even the most deeply entrenched toxins at the cellular level."[275]

Bio-oxidative Therapy using ozone was first used therapeutically during World War I in Germany,[276]England,[277] and France.[278] Today, ozone therapy is restricted by the FDA and made legal only in certain States. Hydrotherapy allows ozone to be delivered via a warm water spray in a spa chamber (under supervision) using dissolved ionized oxygen as O-H water. The heated bath is an aerobic workout that assists the immune system to naturally fight off infections by inducing a slight fever through an increase in body temperature. This stimulates metabolism and the entire cardiovascular system. Raising core body temperature causes perspiration which releases toxins and improves circulation. At therapeutic doses, ozone gas can also be infused into water for drinking, added to an IV solution dripped into the blood, or used as a gas directly into a body orifice (e.g., ear).

The balance of Nature is also expressed by the Redundancy Hypothesis where more than one species will perform a given role within an ecosystem to ensure survival of the whole. When conditions are stressed, if one species disappears, another species increases efficiency to make up the difference in order to maintain stability of the system. The resilience of forest ecosystems is found beneath the soil where trees are symbiotically linked together through networks of fungi.[279] The trees provide carbohydrate energy to the fungi in return for water, carbon, and nitrogen the fungi gather from the Earth. The fungi serve as a pathway of food from nutrient rich "mother" trees to nearby seedlings and younger trees to ensure that balance and stability is maintained in the face of climate change and natural succession.[280] Research shows that the removal of hub trees (clearcutting old growth trees) may compromise the capacity of forests to regenerate.[281]

Physical Regeneration

As Nature teaches, regeneration is the default state of the body. With its neural network that connect mind to heart, heart to brain, and brain to gut, the human body shows us that everything is present for a reason, to sustain the whole. The body's primary effort is to ensure its survival and maintain stasis. The catabolic (breakdown) process and anabolic (buildup) process must be balanced to sustain health.[282] If one kidney fails, the other kidney will increase efficiency to compensate. Inflammation of tonsils, adenoids, lymph nodes, or appendix does not mean they need to be clearcut simply for acting up. Increased activity by some are attempts to compensate for the weakness of others. One for all and all for one. Replenishing a missing element is often all that is needed before balance is restored.

Regeneration is accomplished to protect the heart at all costs, since it is the muscle in the body that never rests. If there is a blockage in the artery highway system, the body is built to simply reroute the flow to prevent a heart attack. Research by Knut Sroka, M.D. shows that the heart creates its own bypass through microcirculation.[283] The increased plaque often observed in arteries is actually a consequence of a heart attack, not the cause. Twenty-four percent of heart attacks are in people without blockages. Therefore, stents and bypass surgery may be unnecessary and may cause more harm than good. Ironically, forcing arteries open through stents causes mircocirculation to collapse.[284] According to Sroka, the cause of heart attack stems from an inability to generate energy at the level of the cell. Instead of oxidative phosphorylation by the mitochondria which generate ATP (energy), there is a shift to the primitive process of glycolysis (fermentation) which leads to lactic acid build-up to cause pain and cramps (i.e., angina in heart, or cramps in leg). This process leads to necrosis of the heart which results in heart attack.[285] If we know that our mitochondria are the synthesis of bacterial and human life then we can surmise some of the reasons why our mitochondria might get sick. The usual suspects include: antibiotics, stress, diabetes, heavy metals, lack of antioxidants, drugs, and statins.

The brain is also capable of regenerating itself, contrary to the belief that once the neural system is formed it is fixed. Like the heart, the brain learns from experience. Any experience, positive or negative causes neurons in the brain to fire. Psychotherapist Linda Graham calls this neuroplasticity. Graham says, "Neurons that fire together many times will wire together." They can form new connections and restructure regions of the brain. Therefore, capacities for coping with stress, which are innate in the brain, develop by experience. If we focus attention and intention on practicing gratitude, empathy, kindness, and compassion, or when we choose our experiences we are causing the neurons to strengthen their connections with each other to create new pathways and to create the brain structure that support those practices. When we develop the structure of the prefrontal cortex of the brain (to make plans and decisions in life), we harness the neuuoplasticity of the brain to become more flexible and more resilient. In a moment of suffering, keeping the mind and heart open to the experience allows you to come out of any overwhelm to be present so you can take the next step with clarity.[286] Graham, who teaches mindfulness practices, recommends long deep (belly) breathing while focusing on the heart to: 1) activate the parasympathetic nervous system to bring the body back into calm, and 2) restore the heart rate to coherence. The research of University of Wisconsin's Neuroscientist Richard Davidson shows that neural connections in the brain can fall apart and rewire by changing beliefs. With compassion and kindness to Self, memories fall apart and rewire to a new sense of Self more in line with our true nature. Because we can choose experiences to rewire the brain, how we cope becomes our responsibility.[287]

Regeneration also happens in utero as the fetus develops. Nature makes it possible for unborn offspring of mammals to regenerate damaged tissue to save their mother's life. Immune cells between mother and fetus are known to move through the placenta to become part of the others' cell line (i.e., michrochimerism). Recent studies of "fetal microchimerism" show that fetal cells have the capacity transfer to the mother to heal maternal tissue damage. These fetal immune cells differentiate into maternal epithelial tissues – thyroid, cervix, intestine and gallbladder,[288] and heart[289] – acting like stem-cells that repair and/or regenerate injured maternal tissues."

When you become tired of counting the ways in which the body is built to regenerate, then go to sleep. Deep sleep is a critical detox-regenerative activity as is evidenced by studies showing that animals begin to die if kept awake for more than six days from hypercatabolism (excess breakdown of tissues).[290] The restorative nature of sleep happens thanks to the newly discovered glymphatic system.[291] The lymphatic system is a detox system of the body as the glymphatic system is the detox system of the brain. The glymphatic system is found in the cerebrospinal fluid and functions at night to clear out waste that has accumulated while awake. During sleep the brain's cells shrink up to sixty percent to allow waste byproducts to pass through more efficiently to the liver to be degraded and recycled. The positive effects of this process, after a nap or a good night's sleep, may cause you to feel as if you have just experienced a brain massage because the dura is cleansed of harmful toxins. Sleep drives metabolic clearance.

According to ancient yogic philosophy, sleep also allows you to unconsciously release identification with the body and merge life force with healing currents in the brain and six spinal centers of the body to recharge with the cosmic energy that sustains all life.

Earthing

Earthing, or grounding, is perhaps the most intimate way to re-Nature, reconnect, and re-synchronize to the natural rhythms. Earthing simply involves taking off your socks and shoes and exposing your bare feet directly to the Earth's surface for healing. The sole of the foot has 1,300 nerve endings per square inch, more than any other part of the body, and is therefore a vital and highly efficient link between the body and the Earth. Every living being that walks the Earth draws energy from the Earth's field through the soles of its feet.

Unlike native cultures, who for thousands of years have understood our energetic or *chi* connection to Mother Earth, we children of technology have all but lost our connection through ignorance. We wear rubber-soled shoes. We connect to the internet. We surround ourselves with high levels of electromagnetic fields (EMFs) that radiate from electronic appliances, computers, cell phones, and cell phone towers.

Our bodies act as antennas to the EMFs, which ground through us and create a surface charge (static electricity) on the body. The closer we are to electrical charges, the greater the negative effects on the body. The most vulnerable time for human exposure to EMFs is during sleep while the body is undergoing recovery, repair, and rejuvenation, when we are in close proximity for many hours to bedroom walls that contain bundled live wires. Therefore, grounding the body becomes important in preventing the effects of overcharging your circuits, which harms the immune system, the nervous system, and every other system of the body. People who fly often, remove themselves from the negative flow of elections from the Earth. One way to reduce or eliminate the effects of jet lag is to immediately ground yourself after a flight and reset your body to earth time.

People who practice Earthing suffer less allergies, inflammation, chronic illness, or flu. In their book *Earthing*, co-authors Ober and Zucker share scientific evidence of restoring the body back to normal physiological patterns when, through Earthing, EMF exposure is neutralized. There are now homeopathic EMF detox formulations as well as grounding mats for city dwellers that can be directly grounded to the earth during sleep to restore head-to-toe electric rhythms to the body as a tool for self-healing.[292] As with any product, do your own research before use.

Primitive Knowledge Rediscovered

At no cost, anyone can stand on the Earth to allow the Earth's flow of electrons to naturally ground the body. Living close to the earth, as ancient Indian cultures knew intimately, is healing to body, mind, and spirit. There is a deep connection between every aspect of the human body and the Earth which sustains it.

The Tarahumara Indians of the Barrancas del Cobre – the copper canyons – of Mexico, described earlier, are a Stone Age tribe of superathletes that, for centuries, have lived on the side of cliffs in the remote wilderness. In his book *Born to Run*, Christopher McDougall describes the Tarahumara as elite runners, noted for their amazing endurance, running forty-eight hours and hundreds of miles without rest to chase down a meal, making it appear effortless. Their agility is matched by their secrecy; not may have seen them in their natural environment. Their superior health and peaceful nature leaves the Tarahumara "immune to the diseases and strife that plague modern existence."[293] Their secret? A deep connection to the Earth, eating native foods and living barefoot. Using the feet in their natural state builds strength. The arch gets stronger under stress and builds elasticity. The barefoot walker or runner allows for a continuous stream of information about the ground and his relationship to it. Adding support by wearing shoes blocks natural movement and weakens the whole structure. The Tarahumara far outpace the best Olympic marathoners in their love of the race.

Native cultures have also known that the length of the hair is an important connection to nature which has been lost to current fashion trends in society. Our perceived need to conform through hairstyles may have come at the expense of connecting to Self. Native Americans and all native cultures leave their hair alone to grow naturally based on tribal beliefs associated with a connection to the ancestors; severing it is a sign of mourning.

A deeper understanding to the purpose of long hair was first revealed during the Vietnam War when native Indian scouts were recruited by government for their 'supernatural' survival instincts and tracking ability. Surprisingly, once enlisted and given a military haircut, the scouts suddenly lost their powers of perception. Their intuition was no longer reliable. They could no longer hear the enemy approaching. "They couldn't 'read' subtle signs as well or access subtle extrasensory information."[294] Further studies verified that it was the length of hair that bestowed these extrasensory abilities. The recruits with long hair kept their stealth.

Long hair, unlike short hair, seems to act as both receiver and transmitter of information as electromagnetic energy, just like our DNA, which negates the argument that it is the hair follicle, not the "dead hair" that is the important focus in the biology of hair.[295] Follicles and hair all work together, just like the sensory nature of a cell. Hair is merely an extension of the body's nervous system that transmits "extra sensory" information – as antennae do – to the brain and chakra systems of the body. Hair is a fractal that functions like a tree sending information through invisible root hairs into the Earth and outward into the atmosphere through its branches, always in communication with its environment.

Another relic of time gone by is found in the Kogi people of Columbia, the last known surviving Native American tribe from the pre-Columbian era. The Kogi society of the Sierra Nevada lives strictly by indigenous spiritual traditions in isolation from the modern world. In complete harmony with Nature, they focus their energy on the inner Self rather than on the body. The Kogi shamens are the sons, the enlightened ones who care for 'Great Mother' their creator, and watch over the community. Like their ancestors of the Tairona culture, the young men spend many years in isolation and darkness to communicate with Spirit 'Aluna' to create harmony and purity in both the spirit and earthly worlds. As the "Elder Brothers" of the planet who see ecological changes in their homeland, they warn us "Younger Brothers" that we must radically change our destructive ways of living if we are to survive.[296]

Science has, only recently, recognized that the seed and the star are the same substance – elements of a single universal consciousness. However, the Dogon of West Africa, a primitive tribe believed to be descended from ancient Egyptians, have celebrated this connection since the thirteenth century. Through spiritual ceremonial rituals and oral tradition that also appear in Sumerian, Babylonian, and Accadian myths, the Dogon tribe knew about the density and orbit of Sirius B, invisible to the naked eye, long before it was confirmed by telescope in 1862[297] and photographed by astronomers in 1970. The secret Dogon technology used to track the cosmos was a germinating seed. The seed represents the creation of life on Earth and all life in the universe. Recent experiments using germinating seeds have confirmed plant consciousness without using electrodes. Using a telescope and sensing equipment, engineer L. George Lawrence and his seeds intercepted signals from the universe.[298] The living seeds lived up to the legend. In receiving a message from the universe, recorded by his equipment, the seeds showed that plants not only communicate with each other, they communicate with all life in the universe.

By the example of the Tarahumara, the Kogi, the Dogon, and Native Americans, we see how we are the Earth and the stars personified. When we own our connection to all life we naturally become responsible guardians of Gaia. Reconnecting with Mother Earth to reach the stars can be as simple as going back to your child self, when you instinctively connected your bare feet to the bare earth on the sand, on the grass, in the mud, and in the water. You didn't know why it felt good, it just did. There were no rules or science about it.

Connecting to the Earth was always an adventure. You didn't realize then that your good health, great sleep, and appetite likely had everything to do with your connection to Nature through your electron exchange from your own bare feet. No matter what was happening inside, you knew where you could find happiness.

A New Breed of Healer

The wisdom of past natural healers like Bernard Jensen, Carey Reams, Max Gerson and others might have been suppressed for a time. Fortunately, in today's digital world, healers are finding innovative ways to push back against a system that prevents choice in the marketplace.

Homeopath Dr. Robert Scott Bell represents a new breed of healer who reaches thousands of people daily and around the world through his nationally syndicated health radio talk show where he teaches a core health-freedom principle: The power to heal is yours. Based on his own healing experience, like so many before him, he offers a dose of wisdom along with healing principles embracing the physical, emotional, mental, spiritual, and political aspects – emphasizing the importance of making informed choices against the onslaught of mixed messages that serve to confuse.

Bell focuses on detoxing the body and restoring integrity to the terrain (gut) as the basis for healing any disease condition. He shares his Silver-Aloe intestinal healing protocol in seminars and on the airwaves without an appointment. The protocol combines the healing benefits of colloidal silver and pure aloe vera juice. Silver has been used for its medicinal and antibiotic properties for thousands of years, since the time of Hippocrates. The ability of a high quality colloidal silver to kill pathogens, control infections, and regenerate tissue in wound healing makes it a natural and safe choice for the body. The aloe carries the silver past the stomach directly into the GI tract, "to achieve the down regulation of inflammation in the gut, while upregulating the healing of tissue,"[299] says Bell. The beauty of this profound protocol lies in its simplicity which serves to cleanse the gut, reverse dysbiosis, and eliminate Candida albacans (yeast) which can no longer find a home (See Bell's Silver-Aloe Intestinal Protocol in Appendix II).

Ignorance has served to keep people thinking that the body is too complex to comprehend and officials have served to keep natural remedies away from the public through suppression and conflicting information. Since nature cannot be patented for profit, no company will spend money to formally test herbs for FDA approval. With FDA as the gatekeeper to approved medicines, natural remedies are made illegal through labeling technicalities and interstate commerce.

Yet, truth shows that natural healing happens through Nature's protocols. Aligning the body with Nature means cleaning up the debris that has accumulated over time and replenishing the nutrients that are missing in action. The body is resilient. And with nature's diversity there is always more than one way to heal. There are as many ways to heal as there are individuals. If anyone tells you there is only their way, turn around and walk the other way. Everyone has an opinion. In a world of opinions there are only consultants.

Some of the most popular natural protocols for reversing disease are plant-based. All plants have a purpose. Ralph Waldo Emerson wrote, "A weed is just a plant whose virtues have not yet been discovered." In many cases, the virtues of plants have been labeled as "weed" and made illegal by government authorities. United States Patent 663057 was initiated in 2003 when researchers discovered that high ratios of cannabinoids found in the marijuana plant had specific healing properties.[300] Cannabinoids naturally bind to receptors throughout the human body, known as the endocannabinoid system, to harmonize and heal. These properties make them useful in a wide range of inflammatory and autoimmune diseases, from neurological insults (stroke, trauma) to neurodegenerative diseases (Alzheimer's and Parkinson's), and cancer, without toxic side effects.

Even as authorities attempt to patent and suppress nature, choosing nutrient-dense, whole, and healthy foods for the body is the way each of us can nurture our ecosystem and be our own healer. We are what we eat – and what we do not eat – since the body will do what it can with what it is given. In healing tumor diseases, from stage 1 to stage 101, there are a myriad of tried-and-true natural modalities that have resulted in hundreds of thousands of people who live to tell about their personal experiences of disease reversal.

All natural therapies have dietary changes at the core. In most cases the first step in reversing disease is to begin with an alkaline diet, which creates a less than optimal environment for tumor cells – a pH above 7.5 – while boosting the immune system. A typical healing diet includes avoiding sugar, dairy, wheat, meat, vegetable oils, corn, soy, eggs, fluoridated-chlorinated water, and alcohol while consuming an excess of raw foods – fresh fruits and vegetables, and vegetable green juices. When the terrain is too alkaline, an acid diet is introduced (meat, fish, dairy, grains, and eggs).

Some of the following dietary protocols make use of a temporary pH shift upward in order to boost the terrain. Alkaline therapy also neutralizes the acid waste of the tumor cells to stop anaerobic fermentation of glucose (tumor cell metabolism) to stop tumor cells from functioning. Other therapies take advantage of nature's ability to select and neutralize pathogens. Common protocols include:

- Hemp or Cannabis oil (Rick Simpson Protocol)
- Moringa Tree Oil
- Ann Wigmore Protocol
- The Gerson Therapy
- The Breuss Organic Vegetable Juice Mix
- Dr. Simonchini's Baking Soda Protocol
- Dr. Berkson's ALA and LDN protocol
- The Budwig Protocol
- Hydrotherapy (ultra-pure oxygenated water) therapy
- Liposomal Vitamin C (antibiotic, antiviral, antihistamine)
- Dr. Burzynski's Antineoplastons (for brainstem glioma)
- Dr. Gonzalas' Individualized Nutrition Protocols

Adjunct therapies include: Herbal blends of Chinese Medicine, Pau D'Arco, apricot kernels, Essiac tea, Chaga Mushroom tea, far infrared, aloe, barley grass, fresh wheat grass juice, MCP, Graviola, kelp (source of iodine), minerals like silica, zinc, selenium, and spices like ginger and cinnamon (anti-inflammatory). (See Suggested Reading List in Appendix III).

The Liver Link

Integral to the renaturing process is liver function. According to traditional Chinese medicine, the center of the soul is found in the liver because the liver is one of the most indispensable organs of detoxification and elimination in the body. In addition to the liver, elimination pathways include the colon, kidneys, skin, lymph, lungs, and brain.

As the main organ system responsible for over five hundred vital functions, the best thing you can do is maintain a fully functional liver to prevent or reverse disease. The body's ability to metabolize anything depends upon the liver. The liver is the gateway to the blood since the liver receives whatever is absorbed by the small intestine via the portal vein before any nutrients flow into the bloodstream. The functions of the liver are to filter toxins from blood and to remove waste by-products so the cells are not damaged and the nervous system can maintain stasis.

Liver, Calcium, pH, and Energy

At the first sign of disease, the liver is the first major organ to take a hit. Any deviation from the ideal cellular pH of 6.4 results in a lack of oxygen in the liver. Without oxygen, the liver cannot pick up calcium to buffer acids within cells. It is the calcium reserve in the body which determines the pH of the tissues, so low calcium levels always cause the pH to drift from 6.4 in either direction. This results in poorer coordination in energy exchange (or frequency) among the liver, blood, and tissues. Your pH is a measure of resistance. Like a speedometer, it shows how fast the energy in your body is moving.

When pH is not optimal, low energy in the liver alters the resistance levels of digestion and leads to a cascade of events in other organs which in turn leads to poor health. When the liver becomes overburdened, contaminants flow back into the blood stream and are recycled to the cells. The ability to receive energy from food is compromised. Free-floating toxins in the blood weaken the nervous system and allow toxins to pass through the blood-brain barrier and affect the mind, causing a person to feel a sense of unease. Someone with a high-functioning liver feels a sense of wellbeing. Likewise, a relaxed person is better able to digest food.

An overloaded liver transfers extra burdens onto accessory organs, including the adrenal glands, which when overloaded contribute to a state of chronic anxiety and tension. The thyroid gland is then called in to assist and becomes first overactive (hyperthyroid) then underactive (hypothyroid) and can toggle between the two states, leading to fogginess and depression. Imbalances in the glands and their hormones contribute to abnormal cell growth which can lead to tumor growth. Tumors are the body's natural way to contain altered, damaged cells in order to eliminate them from the body when the liver has failed. A tumor is nothing more than an acidic, low-oxygen condition of a toxic body.[301]

Knowing the liver's symbiotic relationship with calcium, anyone can correct pH to the right frequency to feed mineral energy to the liver and increase overall energy.[302] Understanding that saliva pH reflects the strength of the liver and the digestive enzyme it produces, it is possible to monitor liver health using a simple saliva pH test in the privacy of your own home and be responsible for your own health. Heal the liver, heal the body, and heal the mind.

THE MIND

Chapter Ten

HEALING THE MIND

"Sometimes people hold a core belief that is very strong. When they are presented with evidence that works against that belief, the new evidence cannot be accepted. It would create a feeling that is extremely uncomfortable, called cognitive dissonance. And because it is so important to protect the core belief, they will rationalize, ignore and even deny anything that doesn't fit in with the core belief."

~Franz Fanon, "Black Skin, White Masks"

Physical Disease Begins in the Mind

"The mind is everything: What you think, you become." This phrase from the Dhammapada, a collection of sayings, is said to originate from the Buddha. It means that the mind is trainable and where you put your energy and thoughts comes to shape the mind. You can either live within the confines of a narrow-mind or you can live laterally, like a Fibonacci spiral.

When it comes to the mind's power, research is showing that over eighty percent of illness – cardiovascular disease, cancer, endocrine and metabolic disease, skin disorders, and infectious ailments – really begins in the mind.[303] The body-mind is inseparable. This is because all negative emotions; worry, fear, anger, bitterness, frustration, grief, temper, depression, self-pity, pride, jealousy, ego, envy, dishonesty, and even excesses such as over-joy, all inhibit the elimination of toxins. The ability to avoid or release stress becomes a major factor in maintaining health.

In the early 1920s, Naturopath Dr. H. Lindlahr wrote in his book *Nature Cure*, "Every thought and every emotion has its direct effect upon the physical constituents of the body. Mental and emotional vibrations become physical vibrations and structures."[304] Negative emotions serve to interrupt the electrical stimulus between the brain and vital organs, especially the liver, where digestive enzymes are weakened. As enzymes fail, mineral deficiencies increase so that even eating a good diet can result in poor absorption and malnutrition. As minerals are depleted, so too is the body's vital force, which is reflected in the symptoms of inflammation and illness. One body feeds the other. Alternatively, emotions of joy, hope, happiness, love, and altruism all correspond to health vibrations. "As a man thinketh, so he is." (Proverbs 23:7). You either control emotions or you allow emotions to control your health.

"Mind is consciousness which has put on limitations. You are originally unlimited and perfect. Later you take on limitations and become the mind."

~Ramana Maharshi, Indian guru (1879–1950)

The Myth of Mental Illness

Like the body, the mind works with what you give it. However, since the mind is not a bodily organ, it cannot be labeled as diseased since the scientific concept of illness refers to a bodily lesion, a material – structural or functional abnormality of the body, as a machine. When it comes to mental illness, Psychiatrist and critic Thomas Szasz M.D. says, "there are no mental diseases, only behaviors of which psychiatrists disapprove and call them "mental illnesses."[305] However, once a mental illness becomes a brain disease – as in the cases of neurosyphilis and epilepsy – then they can be treated. Objective or diagnostic tests that measure physical changes in tissues are different from metaphors that judge behaviors and for which no tests exist (i.e., neurosis and psychoses).

In today's system, whereas patients of most medical practices are voluntary – they choose to be patients – that is not true of psychiatry patients. Under the system, once a person becomes a mental patient, the psychiatrist has the legal right and duty to commit that person to prevent suicide or murder. No other person in society is granted such power of transforming people into patients against their will "and that is the power which psychiatrist much be deprived," says Szasz. In the latest abuses of power, hospitals have quietly begun taking parental rights through transferral of legal guardianship to force hospitalization and chemotherapy on children for alleged experimental research.[306] [307] Author and reporter David Gumpert writes, "Since when did social workers and judges become the arbiters of proper parenting? When did doctors and nurses become the arbiters of which of several possible medical treatments to provide to one's daughter or son in the event of serious illness?"[308]

Before the prohibition of drugs, anyone had the freedom to choose a preferred form of remedy – marijuana, ayahuasca, cannabis, opium, Valium or Haldol – and to decide if the drug worked or not. Patients had the option of seeking out holistic physicians to reverse disease. However, since psychiatry came into being, choice has become medicalized. Currently, the only option for someone labeled "mental" is pharmaceutical drugs. The only route to these drugs is through licensed physician under a lucrative business model with laws that make prescription drugs legal and everything else illegal. Because the ability to choose a drug should be a fundamental human right, similar to choosing books, prayer, or forms of exercise, Szasz believes all prescription laws and drugs laws should be repealed and abolished.

Filmmaker, Kevin P. Miller in his documentary film *Generation Rx* reveals that over the last two decades, mood-altering drugs have become the fastest growing class of drugs in the world targeting our kids, with annual sales in the billions of dollars. Ten million kids are labeled without diagnostic tests and prescribed psychotropic drugs because parents have been convinced by doctors, by schools, and by the media that our children's brains are biological defects that can only be controlled by chemicals. What is not disclosed is that these drugs block normal systems of judgment, cause biochemical and nutrient imbalances, and create the negative effects of weight gain, autoimmune diseases, brain atrophy, violence, and, in some cases, suicide as the brain naturally attempts to compensate. Miller says, "It is a chemical manipulation of consciousness without regard for human life."

The disease label ADHD (attention deficit hyperactivity disorder) is, in fact, the cause created by the companies that also provide the drug-based "cure" (i.e., Ritalin ®) to boost profit margins. In his last interview, seven months before his death, American psychiatrist Leon Eisenberg, known as the scientific father of ADHD is quoted as saying: "ADHD is a prime example of a fictitious disease." Eisenberg had earlier described this condition as a "hyperkinetic reaction of childhood."[309]

In France, kids are not diagnosed with ADHD because French psychiatrists don't attribute all symptoms to a biological dysfunction of the child's brain. Their holistic approach allows for considering nutritional causes for ADHD symptoms – "specifically the fact that the behavior of some children is worsened after eating foods with artificial colors, certain preservatives, and/or allergens."[310] Recent studies now show that symptoms of children diagnosed with ADHD stem from nutrition deficit disorder (NDD) – lack of important minerals (zinc, copper),[311] neurotoxic effects of food dyes,[312] agents that induce hyperkinetic behavior,[313] – and can be controlled through diet [314] [315]

If balance in body, mind, and spirit represents true power, then the effect of one group (psychiatrists) purposely shackling the spirit of another group (children) through drugs is nothing short of medical slavery. Author and presenter Graham Hancock says, "There is a war on consciousness in our society and if we as adults are not allowed to make sovereign decisions for what to experience with our own consciousness while doing no harm to others, including the decision to use responsible ancient and sacred plants, then we cannot claim to be free."[316]

The truth is that anything can be the cause of emotional problems defined as "mental," from being poor to being wealthy to being cast out of society – anything that creates distress. The current profit-based system would rather label the problem a disease than attempt to bring the person back into balance. Whereas three centuries ago sickness, poverty, suicide, and war were seen as religious problems (witchcraft could get you burned at the stake), today they are all seen as medical, psychiatric problems, curable with therapy. Due to political and educational dumbing down, not many people have noticed the insidious and subtle transformation that has taken place. In the church of scientism, doctors can declare that your genes cause everything from what ails you to whether or not you will survive marriage.[317]

The Gene Theory… Is Only a Theory

Western Medicine has long claimed that our genes predetermine our body-mind health. Science claims that your disease is written in our DNA to reveal itself at some future point in time. Yet if disease is encoded in our genes, why then doesn't disease reveal itself at birth? And why would only a select few "experts" hold the key to your DNA when your genetic code has been passed down over the centuries specifically to you?

If doctors could read your DNA like a crystal ball, perhaps they could develop a custom made drug so you have less of a risk of getting divorced in a country where there are now more unmarried than married couples. That is exactly what the Human Genome Project (HGP) hoped to provide when it launched in 1998 – the key to unlocking all the answers. With its conclusion in 2003, the project failed to find the expected 100,000 genes believed necessary to encode the same number of proteins known to be present in the body. Only 20,000-25,000 genes were discovered, roughly the same number as the roundworm.

In putting the cart before the horse, the blueprint model of genetics – one gene $\rightarrow$ one protein $\rightarrow$ one cellular behavior – failed to tell the complete story of the human being. While the conclusions have never officially been made public, the project has been criticized by some who say the premise failed to account for cultural and environmental differences, and others who say it could be used to discriminate against people. Ethical questions have also been raised about the lack of meaningful consultation with the indigenous groups that were the subjects of the study.[318] The assumption that the nucleus of each cell provides the roadmap for life and health has never been scientifically proven in the first place.

What the HGP did reveal is that genes are the blueprints for proteins, not the blueprints for life. Genes make protein for cells. Like any architect's blueprint, genes do not self-activate. A gene cannot turn itself on or off just like a balloon cannot blow itself up. Only a signal from the environment can make that happen, can activate an expression of a gene. Your nervous system controls the reading and modifying of the blueprint. Genes aside, when it comes to getting along with your mate, finding bliss may simply reflect the fact that the institution of marriage has become obsolete in light of the freedom gained in the art of cohabitation.

As we have begun to explore the untapped ninety-seven percent of our brain, the Gene Theory is quickly being replaced with a more intuitive model of the cell where *epigenetic* factors – beyond the control of the gene – determine how DNA will be expressed. In other words, our DNA itself does not determine our behavior. Rather, our cells express themselves based on environmental stimuli which activate our genes, turning them on or off like a switch.

Epigenetics

Western allopathic medicine maintains that genetics are the main factor in predisposing someone to disease, with very little emphasis on the effects of diet. Yet Nature shows the opposite, that food choices protect against disease to which our genes may predispose us. Epigenetics – epi meaning "beyond" – shows how our surroundings and our perceptions are more powerful and influential to health than we realize, and that both our environment and our beliefs alter our DNA, which are passed on to future generations right along with eye color.

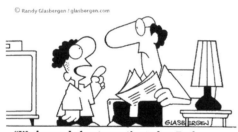

"We learned about genetics today, Dad. I inherited your eye and hair color. I also inherited your memories of Wild Susie and the summer of '68!"

In his book *Biology of Belief*, author and Cell Biologist Bruce Lipton challenges conventional wisdom when he reveals that the brain of the cell is not actually the nucleus as we have been taught to believe. The cell membrane, the skin of the cell, is really the brain; think mem-brain. Lipton's experiments showed that if the nucleus is removed from the cell, the cell continues to function for two or more months completely unaffected. The cell continues to communicate with other cells, eats, grows, eliminates waste, recognizes toxins and food, and goes about its life until the proteins break down. Indeed, genes do not control biology because the cell exhibits normal behavior patterns without them. The nucleus is not present for intelligence, only as the blueprint for making proteins.[319] By his efforts

Lipton took a risk. But in doing so he opened a new awareness to many in the physical sciences.

The nucleus as all-powerful had been an assumption, never scientifically proven. Lipton had noted that both the cell membrane and the human brain derive from a germ layer called the ectoderm. Until Lipton, no one thought to pursue the significance of this connection. But in looking beyond, he further revealed that when stem cells (genetically identical cells) were placed in different petri dishes with different culture fluids, they differentiated into different cells (fat, muscle, or bone cells), just as fetal cells are able to differentiate in the womb. Likewise, if cells were placed in a nutrient deficient environment, they got sick. When the environment (culture medium) was changed, they improved.

Like the lining of the gut and the skin of our body, the cell membrane is the interface between the cell's inner and outer environments. The cell membrane takes an environmental stimulus – sun, air, sound, chemical, smell, taste – and converts it into a secondary signal that controls a protein in the cell membrane. That signal activates a specific behavior inside the cell. The behavior is mediated by the cell membrane as it responds to its environment. In this way, the cell's behavior is not programmed but is continually responding to the environmental stimulus, adjusting and adapting as needed. In essence, the membrane is a switch.[320] The new paradigm of the cell reinforces our place in Nature. Looking at the big picture, or the microscopic one, we see that we are our environment. There is no separation.

One strikingly sweet example of environmental influence on our genes is a nutritional study from Australia[321] showing that a one-off sugar hit affects human cells for a two-week period by switching off genetic controls designed to protect the body against diabetes and heart disease. In diabetics who have extended periods of high blood glucose, arterial damage persists long after insulin therapy reduces their man glucose levels. Even if we don't want to know that sugar is bad for us, our cells remember. When cells see sugar, they alter natural metabolic responses (i.e., trigger histone modifications) and replicate those effects on the body, almost as if they have been coerced to lower defenses and go against their sworn orders. Not only that, but bad eating habits prolong the effects of sugar to permanently alter DNA.

Genetically-altered grains and produce are additional hazards in the American food supply even as many countries ban genetically modified organisms (GMOs) based on deleterious health effects. The new GMO wheat creates proteins in the wheat engineered to turn off genes permanently. Since these genes match human genes, these molecules potentially silence our genes if ingested. Not only can they redirect human DNA to make proteins the body has never before seen, but these genes become incorporated into the skin and digestive tract to be passed down to future generations and integrated into the human genome. The toxicity of the poison is amplified in plants and animals with immune responses to foods that were previously harmless, because each cell now contains its own pesticide "spray bottle."[322][323] In the United States, GMOs are considered proprietary information and are not labeled when sold in stores so people cannot make informed decisions about what they eat.[324]

Epigenetics reflects the normal functioning of our genes. It tells us that the ability for food to prevent or cause disease now has a basis in science. It provides us with proof that the human body is really a complex ecosystem, dependent upon and interconnected with its environment.

Cellular perceptions at the microscopic level reflect our beliefs at the macroscopic level. Based on his experiments, Lipton suggests that we not only adjust our genes to fit the environment we live in but we adjust our genes based on the environment we *think* we live in. Thoughts – how we think and what we think – become a critical factor in health. Not only does perception activate behavior and activate genes, but it can also rewrite genes. At the level of our whole Self, it is really our beliefs that select our genes and our behavior, which includes our thoughts and our emotions.

As reflected by the life of each cell, our lives are based on how we respond to our environment, how we see the signals – our perception – and then how we convert those signals into a response. Awareness of the environment through physical sensation equals perception.

In his book *The Spontaneous Healing of Belief*, author Gregg Braden writes, "…the experience of our lives is based on a program – a reality code – that translates possibilities into reality. Belief is that code. If we know how to create the right kind of belief, then our ideas of what 'is' and 'isn't' change forever. In other words, nothing is impossible in a world based in belief."[325]

"If you believe that you can or you believe that you can't, you're right."

~Henry Ford, founder of Ford Motor Company

The Stress Reaction

Everyone is exposed to stressors. However, it is a choice in how we respond to those stimuli that determines our quality of health. If we choose to become "stressed out," one of the first physical reactions is that our breathing becomes shallow. Shallow breathing reduces the amount of oxygen to our lungs, cells, and body, which leads to inflammation. When stress is ongoing, inflammation becomes chronic. Over time, inflammatory molecules can cross the blood-brain barrier to cause apathy, fatigue, and changes in eating habits.

Under stress, the fight-or-flight response kicks in and the adrenals become exhausted. The body cannot relax and has trouble sleeping. Lack of sleep prevents the body from rebuilding, repairing, and rejuvenating by impairing the glymphatic "garbage disposal" system of the brain. Excess waste in the body further taxes the adrenals, which pump up adrenaline production. Increased adrenaline causes the body to step up metabolism to quickly boost energy for the body. The pituitary gland increases its production of adrenocorticotropic hormone (ACTH), which stimulates the release of the hormones cortisone and cortisol. These hormones inhibit disease-fighting white blood cells and further suppress the immune response.

Stress also increases the level of the protein interleukin-6 (IL-6), which has direct effects on most of the cells in the body. Digestion slows or stops, absorption slows, fats and sugars are released from stores in the body, and

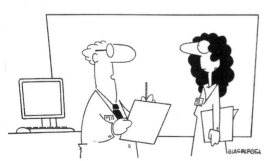

Copyright 2006 by Randy Glasbergen.
www.glasbergen.com

"According to my research, laughter is the best medicine, giggling is good for mild infections, chuckling works for minor cuts and bruises, and snickering only makes things worse."

the viscosity of the blood changes slightly, making it more likely for blood to clot.

In reacting to stress, you always have a choice. You can choose to take antidepressants to artificially numb the underlying emotions that will continue to rise up. Or you can choose to see the sunny side of life and laugh at your mistakes. You can allow emotions to control you or you can take control of your emotions. Knowing how your perceptions alter your very biology should help you appreciate the miracle you are. If you know the power of your words, thoughts, and beliefs, you have all the tools you need to make healthy adjustments.

The Power of Words

The word "cancer" elicits a sense of fear that permeates the body and can be more lethal than the cancer itself, increasing the risk of death from both suicide and cardiovascular causes.[326] When we picture cancer as an uncontrolled growth of cells, this image clouds our perception so that the rational mind shuts down. The same holds true for false positive breast screenings, which can result in depression, dejection, and an inability to sleep.[327] When patients see themselves as victims they become victims.

Spiritual teachers have long known that the body responds to language and thoughts. This is because your DNA's genetic code follows the same basic grammar and syntax rules as all human languages. The great discovery of this century reveals that human language is a direct reflection of our own DNA. Your DNA does not have to be decoded or spliced to understand it. DNA needs no fixes. DNA naturally responds to language when the proper vibrations (or sound frequencies) are used.

This discovery was first made in 1990 by Russian scientists who proved that DNA can be reprogrammed simply through words and thoughts. Russian biophysicist and molecular biologist Pjotr Garjajev and his colleagues at the Russian Academy of Science in Moscow found the DNA spiral to be an oscillating electromagnetic antenna that not only stores information but also receives, transmits, and further interprets it. While the Human Genome Project was focused on five percent of the encoding triplets of DNA, Garajajev's experiments studied the whole human genome.

By stepping back to look at the larger picture, Garjajev discovered that our DNA is not merely a static code but rather a living, reprogrammable software package that responds to language-modulated laser rays and even to radio waves, if the proper frequencies are used.[328] [329] In fact, only ten percent of our DNA is used for making proteins.

Just as crystals are able to hold, store, and release light energy, our own DNA corresponds to a biological internet in that it reacts to energy whether that energy is language[330] or thoughts or emotion or whether it is the energy of the food we eat. This concept scientifically explains the phenomenon of clairvoyance, intuition, and self-healing. In other words, healing happens on a subatomic level.

In metaphysical terms, our bodies are electric and magnetic. Each cell, like each mineral or crystal, vibrates at a unique frequency determined by the ratio of its subatomic particles (protons, neutrons, and electrons). Looking deeper into these particles, we realize there are no particles at all, only vortices of energy, similar to the essence of a homeopathic remedy. What appears to be physical is really an illusion from energy.

Reality is Relative

Our eyes have been deceiving us all along. According to quantum physics, matter does not exist with certainty in any one place but instead shows "tendencies" to exist. It changes between particles and waves depending on when it is being observed. Our world of solid objects is 99.99999999 percent empty space. It is really a world of wave-like patterns of interconnections and more specifically, probabilities of interconnections.[331] That means the book you're holding, the screen you are viewing, the chair you're sitting on, and you are mostly not there. Nothing is set in stone. Even a stone on your path is merely a probability. The universe is not random and not predictable. It is mutable, ever-changing, a dynamic web of energy patterns intermingling to form a whole. We, as creative observers, are strands within this web and as such, reflect and affect everything around us. A shift of one affects the whole web.

"Whether you observe a thing or not depends on the theory which you use. It is the theory that decides what can be observed."

~Albert Einstein, theoretical physicist

Einstein's Theory of Relativity $E = mc^2$ published in 1905, describes the equivalence relationship of mass and energy such that mass (m) can be changed into energy (E) and vise versa with the speed of light constant.

Einstein theorized that the particle and the wave are not separate at all. After his equation was taken by others and manifested into the detonation of the atomic bomb in Japan, one of Einstein's last acts was to sign a public declaration calling on world leaders to renounce all war. What scientists understood only after Einstein's death is that $E = mc^2$ is not only the equation of destruction but also the ultimate equation of creation.[332] In essence, mass and energy are interchangeable. Mass is just one form of energy.

When we describe our physical biology in terms of the science of epigenetics and our new understanding of relativity we see that Darwin did not have it exactly right when he suggested that evolution is based on random selection. In fact, if you do not posses the appropriate genes to respond to a stressful stimulus, your cells will chemically induce a mutation to occur in what is known as *adaptive mutation*. This is not a random act since the environment controls the mutation and the mutation is environmentally directed in favor of life.

At the level of the cell it is the cell membrane that is the true brain. The cell "mem-brain" identifies what from its environment will be allowed in and what will be kept out. Since epigenetic, not genetic factors, are primary in determining disease outcome, we are not victims of our genes. We no longer have the excuse to blame our problems on our inheritance. On the other hand, our genes may be victims of our self-perception. Suddenly, what we believe and how we see things becomes critically important to life. It explains why a group of ten people who witness a car accident will relate ten different accounts of what happened. It describes why Pasteur saw the germ and deduced one thing while his counterparts, Bernard and Bechamp saw shapeshifters and deduced another. Everyone is seeing, or not seeing, his own truth take shape as waves and particles.

Thomas Young (1773-1829) an English physician, professor of physics, and Renaissance man of the early nineteenth century, first demonstrated this particle-wave effect in his double-slit experiment which not only went against Isaac Newton's theory that light is only a particle.

Young showed that matter and energy display characteristics of both particles and waves, and that the mere act of watching affects the results.[333]

For more than a century, quantum mechanics used measurement devices showing that light is present as either a particle or a wave. However, recently physicists at the University of Bristol have confirmed, using a new device called a quantum photonic chip, that particle-wave duality occurs simultaneously. For the first time since 1801 when Young first conducted his experiment, proof now exists that a particle can be many places at the same time. In fact, it can be in infinitely many places at the same time, just like a wave.

"Everything we call real is made of things that cannot be regarded as real."

~Niels Bohr, theoretical physicist

The "Observer Effect" is now a fundamental scientific premise of quantum theory as defined by Physicist Niels Bohr, who recognized that reality is really a set of possibilities and probabilities of relationships, and that things do not come into being until an observer observes them. The very act of observation affects the thing being observed. In other words, the nature of matter depends on *whether* one looks, and the *way* the one looks. The idea that the observer is not separate from the object observed goes back to Advaita Vedanta, a school of ancient Vedic philosophy which teaches that everything starts from the inside and moves out. Theoretical Nuclear Physicist, Amit Goswami sums it up like this: "Quantum physics enables us to see directly that we can make sense of the world only if we base the world on consciousness."

Theoretical physicist David Bohm and Neurophysiologist Karl Pribram separately described reality as a *holographic universe* in which we are not separated parts of a whole. The cell membrane is a hologram of the same mechanism acting between the human body and its own environment. Every piece of the hologram in the universe is an exact representation of the whole and as such, each piece can reconstruct the entire image. We are a whole. We are our environment. As above so below. The microcosm is the Macrocsm. The body is a symbol of something greater.

Quantum physicist, Dr. William A. Tiller's studies and experiments have shown that human consciousness changes space, and that the mind affects matter. Tiller demonstrated this by imprinting a pH device with an intention to either raise or lower the pH of water. He then shipped the device to a separate location where it was placed near the target jar of water and turned on. Not only was the pH seen to change by 1.5 full units (more than ten-fold), but when the experiment was repeated over and over, the room became conditioned and the effect happened more quickly each time. Eventually the pH change would happen when the device was no longer in the room. Tiller defined a zero point energy field or vacuum of potential energy that is amorphous and can be accessed and altered through human intent.[334]

In other words, the state of the particles that make up physical reality can be changed. Tiller's experiment presents a solid scientific basis that concrete reality comes from the interaction between consciousness and matter. Things in life always come from the choice of possibilities. He believes the power of our future lies in harnessing this zero point field of potential, the space between the atoms, cells, stars, planets, galaxies, and whole universes.

Chapter Eleven

EVERYTHING IS ENERGY

The reason that our perceptions and beliefs affect us down to our cells is because everything is vibrating energy. Thoughts are energy and cells are energy. They are electromagnetic realities. Thoughts are translated by the nervous system and affect each cell's behavior. It is not a stretch of the imagination to believe what Einstein, Garajajev, Tiller, Tolle, Lipton, and Chopra each suggest through their own innovations and discoveries: That if we can shift thought energy, we alter the behavior of our cells. It is not mind *over* matter but mind *into* matter.

What you learned in science class is not the whole story. Your cells are not solely programmed by your DNA because you are not a machine. Instead, your cells continually respond to environmental signals – including thoughts, language, and emotions – and adjust moment by moment. Every word and every thought has its own vibration, which affects every bone, muscle, and cell in the body, each with its own vibration. This explains why affirmations and hypnosis with heart-based feeling can be so powerful in changing behavioral patterns. If you change one belief then the whole web vibrates in a new rhythm.

"We do not 'come into' this world; we come out of it, as leaves from a tree. As the ocean 'waves,' the universe 'peoples.' Every individual is an expression of the whole realm of nature a unique action of the total universe."

~Alan Watts, "The Book on the Taboo on Knowing Who You Are

125

Every day you experience how the mind-body connection works on a primal level when your mouth begins to water and digestive juices begin to flow as you think about, see, or smell food. Your heart beats faster when you see or think about someone you love. Every thought and every feeling resonates and influences every cell of your body. Therefore it is not difficult to accept that an optimistic state of mind creates a healthy body and a pessimistic or depressed state of mind generates metabolic changes that invite dis-ease.

The term energy is reflective of a resistance to a vibration because energy is only measurable through resistance. There is a vibration, and that which resists the vibration, which manifests as heat, electricity, thought, belief, emotion, etc. Without resistance there is pure flow. Energy master Michael Monk says, "As most of matter is empty space, we are the empty space through which it all flows."[335]

The Chakra System

E-motion equals energy in motion. Emotional energy in the form of anger, grief, sadness, fear, or jealousy not only block elimination pathways of the liver and other organs, they also block energetic pathways of the energy body known as the *chakra system.*

The chakra system is described by ancient Buddhist and Vedic teachings as energy from the universal energy field flowing into the body through energy centers called chakras (wheels of light). Seven primary chakras lie along your spine and are located at major endocrine gland sites. It is no accident that the chakras align with the glands, which are the guardians of wellbeing. Each system reflects energy rhythms; the chakras move universal energy, the glands secret and move biochemical hormones. The hormones modulate the emotions. Understanding the endocrine-chakra connection leads us to see the relationship between color, light, hormones, and emotions as one.

Secondary chakras are energy centers located at junctures of bone, joint, and a nerve plexus. As each chakra spins it generates its own electromagnetic field in a unique color, each combining to create your aura (the eighth chakra). The higher the amount of energy produced by a particular chakra, the more dominant its color in the aura. Someone in a state of high emotion – fear or "fight, flight, or freeze" – will show an orange (second chakra) aura reflecting activated adrenal glands, while someone in a highly creative state will generate a blue (fifth chakra) aura, equating to an activated thyroid.[336]

The chakra system is a central processing center for every aspect of your personality and sensibilities in the same way your glands represent various centers of the immune system. The fourth chakra (heart chakra) is the center of the seven primary chakras, identified as the astral body, between the lower planes (physical, emotional, mental) and the higher planes (etheric, celestial, ketheric) of the energy body. Its location reflects a bridge between the dimensions of matter and spirit. The heart chakra also contains the thymus gland which is the neurological center of the immune system.

All living things including the Earth, the sun, and all planets, are interconnected to each other and to the greater whole through universal energy. Like the human body, Earth embodies her own chakra system or energy grid made up of "ley lines," or spiritual pathways, mapped by ancient surveyors that encircle the Earth equidistant from each other. They can be easily identified using a dousing rod. These energy currents, or fields were critical to ancient Indian and Egyptian cultures as fertile agricultural sites and to important structures like the pyramids of Giza.

"If you wish to find the secret of the universe, think of energy, frequency, and vibration."

~Nikoa Tesla, inventor, physicist, engineer

Universal energy flows into and out of each human chakra as a vortex, like funnels or whirlpools, and also flows from the Earth through your feet to the higher energy centers and out the crown of your head. It also flows in reverse from above through the crown chakra. These points of energy radiate outward along twelve meridians on each side of the body. Chinese Medicine postulates that meridians are made up of water clusters, each cluster possessing a positive charge on one side and a negative charge on the other. These clusters link up like a chain along the meridians and when they move they emit electromagnetic energy, which becomes a component of external chi.[337] When meridians are blocked, chi does not circulate, the body loses balance, and we become ill. The goal is to have all chakras activated and open to the flow so that the endocrine system is balanced for physical health and energy is balanced for emotional, and metaphysical health.

As energy healers, we each become an open channel to universal energy. When we are open, there is no resistance. We are able to transmute Earth plane energy to spiritual energy and spiritual energy into Earth-plane energy through the heart (fourth chakra). We can send this energy distantly to others or to ourselves. As the body heals itself we learn that we are each healers by birthright. As energy workers we facilitate the remembering of our true selves whether energy healing is done in person or distantly.

The aura of light in each person is an actual rainbow of color and represents our energetic connection to the realm of pure consciousness; our essence. This light body emits light waves in the invisible infrared range to the full spectrum range to ultraviolet range. These emissions are similar to those of radio stations. The aura carries information that is measurable, especially along fingertips, as surface electrical tension. An average person emits 50-100 millivolts. Healthy children emit 200 millivolts. Qigong masters and psychics are known to emit 20,000 millivolts or higher.[338]

Though we all connect to the same universal energy system, we are each unique. Therefore, each chakra spins and spirals differently within the body, day to day. The aura and chakra system is a force field with a thumbprint. It is an energy pattern that carries our memories and life story. It is who we are at our core.

By appreciating the connection between our auric layers, our chakras, and our physical body as one, we as artists gain greater insight of our true abilities. It is another opportunity to see with new eyes where disease originates and how body-mind and spirit are always working together to find balance to heal the whole.

Our chakras filter environmental energies which pass from the mind of the higher self to the conscious mind, as thoughts. These thoughts flow to us based on our individual belief systems to guide our actions. Simply by observing the consequences of our actions, we should be able to identify whether we've chosen a beneficial belief system or not. We can simply become the observer of the movie of our life, knowing that we are also the writer, producer, and actor. As creatures of Nature, working with the universal Law of Attraction, we see how we attract like situations and like-minded friends based on our belief systems. Anything contrary will inform us that we are not "on track."

When we find ourselves constantly facing emotional difficulties, we end up reacting to their electromagnetic realities in our physical experience. If we always push against situations or people, we will tend to create more of the same. What you resist persists. In these situations, we are not directing life but reacting to it. Fortunately, the opposite is also true. What you allow flows to you.

Author Hermann Hesse wrote in his work, Siddhartha, "The river is everywhere." If he is correct then the easiest way to travel is to go with the flow. As artists, we must see that these experiences are visuals or living paintings of our inner beliefs. If you don't like what you see, then try changing the visual in your mind. Too often our suppressed or limiting beliefs end up blocking the flow of inner energy flowing outward. In distorting the flow of energy, we throw off our vital force and eventually the physical body.

Under chronic stress, chakras can reverse spin, slow down, or stop completely. As a consequence, the flow of energy is kept from being released through the crown chakra. Stuck energy is stored in the body and will vibrate to a specific organ system. Anger and frustration migrate to the liver and gallbladder. Fear and anxiety seek out the bladder and kidneys. Loss of power or responsibility goes to the pancreas. Lack of joy goes to thyroid. Excess in any form goes to the heart. A blockage in one chakra will create a state of low chi in multiple chakras, which often includes the heart or the blood. A weak energy field weakens the physical body by blocking the elimination of toxins.

Louise Hay's books describe the connection between disease symptoms and their negative mental influences, along with countering affirmative thought re-patterns. In her book, *You Can Heal Your Life*, Hay suggests that nearsightedness stems from a fear of seeing one's future and of not trusting what lies ahead in life. Nearsightedness can result from something the person did not want to see on an emotional, psychological or spiritual level. By changing words and thoughts the body changes. Changing thought patterns can bring clarity.

Naturopathy, homeopathy, acupuncture, acupressure, therapeutic/healing touch, reflexology, chakra balancing, reiki, qigong, craniosacral therapy, meditation, yoga, emotional freedom technique

(EFT), tension releasing exercises (TRE), crystal healing, and others are all natural healing tools that balance the energy body to enhance self-healing. They unscramble the blocks of the biofield to allow energy to flow in the correct direction and at the correct speed to reverse disease.

There are many ways to access the body's self-healing tools. Rupert Sheldon, the creator of Matrix Energetics, uses the concept of the morphic field to describe the collective consciousness, which is accessed through the heart rather than the head. Matrix Energetics recognizes that because everything is comprised of patterns of light and information, anyone can reprogram negative emotions and rewrite thoughts. By breaking through the matrix, you reactivate your electrical circuits to change physical outcomes.

TRE (tension releasing exercises) pioneered by David Berceli, Ph.D., is a self-administered protocol to release deep, chronic tension to restore balance. TRE is uses simple, painless exercises to release chronic muscle contractions that remain in the body created by severe shock, stress, anxiety, or trauma. Tension is trapped in the psoas muscle, the powerful center of the body that connects the back, legs, and pelvis. When this high state of aroused energy is prevented from being eliminated, it remains trapped in a bio-neural-physiological loop that will continue to repeat a pattern of protection and defense in an attempt to fully discharge the energy. TRE evokes the psoas muscle to tremor which reverberates throughout the entire body to naturally dissolve deep tension. As the energy from the psoas is released, it signals the body to return the body to a state of rest and recuperation.

The ho'oponopono process is a Hawaiian method used as a clearing meditation that releases memories or programs that we have recorded in our subconscious. An appeal for atonement and forgiveness is made in order to correct and heal thoughts and memories that hold us back. The meditation uses breathing and a mantra: I am sorry. Please forgive me. I love you. Thank you. It is love that first neutralizes the emotions that caused the problem and then love that releases the neutralized emotions from the thoughts, leaving you open so that the healing light of love can fill the void.[339]

Crystals have been used in ancient cultures as energetic healing tools since they amplify the power of intention. They also metabolize universal life force energy to a form the body can digest and use for its spiritual growth.[340] Crystals are divided into seven groups for identification based on their geometric formation, growth pattern, and symmetry. Each group in color also corresponds to the seven chakra systems based on their individual frequencies.

The various healing modalities evidence that there is no one-way to heal. Healing happens not only in the natural world for the physical body, but also in the spiritual realm for the mental, emotional, and spirit bodies. All three aspects are healed together or they are not healed for long. Healing the whole Self means taking care of the body and also freeing ourselves from unconscious beliefs and implicit biases.

Psychologist Eldon Taylor says our implicit biases related to race, sex, and age predetermine our expectations and causes us to see what is not there. The checkerboard effect is an example of how our collective biases frame our reality. We believe the squares alternate as black and white when they are side by side, when in reality they are all the same shade of gray. Is it a trick of the eye or an implicit bias that creates the expectation of different shades? Taylor says it is the bias that determines what we see.[341]

Whether using hypnosis, meditation, or any of healing techniques described above, all serve to bring awareness to our biases, assumptions, and patterns of belief. Only when we are aware of them can we let them go. This letting go of self-limiting beliefs is important in creating the energetic space to take action on the new belief. By changing a belief, you shift your vibration and in turn shift the vibration for the collective web.

"There are no obstacles that can't be used as stepping stones."

~Dr. Bernard Jensen, N.D.

One effect of a shift is that you begin to attract new experiences and people into your life who resonate with your new frequency. By being clear about what you don't want, you discover what you do. When you reject what no longer serves you, you create healthy boundaries. You lift yourself up emotionally, spiritually, and physically. You revive your vital force. You recover your health. No one else does this for you; it's all you.

When you are firmly grounded in who you are and your place in the universe, it means your solar plexus located at your third chakra is open and healthy. From the third, one finds spiritual wisdom and a sense of belonging. Since this light center is your "seat of power" it is related to the mind. A healthy third chakra means you are able to overcome inherent weaknesses and obstacles because you stop over thinking and over analyzing. You develop your innate power to find your own answers. And as you open and clear the higher chakras, you can't help but achieve greater spiritual awareness.

Understanding Your Chakras

The spin of your chakras can be indirectly observed by placing a pendulum above each one to see the energy as it rotates the pendulum.

Chakra System

Number	Name/Location	Character	True Color
7	Crown of head	Totality of Beingness. Spiritual Perfection	Violet
6	Forehead (3rd eye)	Visualization. Clairvoyance	Indigo
5	Thyroid	Communication. Creative Expression	Blue
4	Heart	Universal love. Compassion. Empathy	Green
3	Solar Plexus	Creation of Self. Perception/Projection Seat of emotions. Personal power.	Yellow
2	Sacral (pubic)	Desire, including sexual energy	Orange
1	Base of spine	Physical vitality. Survival. Security	Red

Balancing Male and Female Energy

Each of us can become blocked at any one chakra or at multiple chakras. Any block represents an imbalance within. When we fail to voice an opinion or continually stop ourselves from speaking our truth, the fifth chakra (throat chakra) will become blocked. Using a pendulum to douse the qualities of your chakras can show the spin of the vortex. The circumference of the vortex will be shallow or wide, reflecting how open or closed the chakra is.

Today thyroid disease and thyroid cancer are the fastest growing disorders around the world, primarily among women. Thyroid disease represents an iodine deficiency of the physical body. The physical manifests from the energetic, suggesting most women women fail to use their voices. Perhaps they fail to express themselves in favor of keeping the peace, or because they believe they have nothing to offer. Men commonly suffer from heart disease. The physical heart can suffer from mineral deficiencies. A fourth chakra blockage, however, also reveals an inability to give and receive love in a relationship. Men tend to put up walls around their hearts for protection from the fear of being hurt.

In order to come into balance, we cannot be looking for an opposite to complete us. Men need to open to the vulnerability of their feminine side. Women need to open to the strength of their masculine side. Each must expose both sides – sensitivity and power – courage and compassion, practicality and spirituality--from within before true balance can be gained.

Perhaps at the core of our emotional deficiencies, we are not using our gifts out of fear. All fear-based behaviors prevent us from expressing who we are. Any fear is limiting to full health and success. It leads to depression, apathy, and feeling "stuck." A fear about what someone else thinks about you weakens the thymus and reduces the body's ability to move toxins out for healing. It is the heart chakra that boosts your immunity. Love heals.

To demonstrate this, researchers measured feelings of appreciation, compassion, and love as a smooth, rolling "coherent" heart rhythm, while feelings of anger, frustration, and fear produced a jagged "incoherent" image. These heart rhythms lead to chemical, electrical, neurological, and hormonal changes in the body. It is not the heart rate in beats per minutes but the specific rhythm, the time period *between* two heartbeats that determine the outcome between disease and health.[342] The saying "a change of heart changes everything" is now verifiable using an electroencephalogram (EEG) and biofeedback with meditation. Other research shows those who both give and receive the most compassionate love while maintaining compassionate love towards self (related to self-worth and self-forgiveness) have substantially less disease progression based on CD4 cell count, a reflection of the strength of the immune system.[343]

Feelings of love lead to increases in the hormone DHEA to prevent aging, while stress and depression lead to increases in cortisol to bring about aging. This resonance has an observable ripple effect on people nearby. The positive energy of a laugh or a smile can be just as contagious as the negative energy of a glare or an insult. Love and fear are both emotional states that affect our immediate environment and our physical health. What we believe matters and becomes matter. When we believe we are victims of our environment, we are and forever will be. Change has to come from within before we see and experience it without. Letting go of stress, and more importantly the fear behind the stress, boosts the immune system.

Knowledge equals the power to heal. Knowing your power to control your stress level by slowing your breathing and changing your thoughts, changes your reality. Knowing the physical *and* energetic causes of your dis-ease puts you in control. Spending a few minutes managing your emotions by meditating or shifting your thoughts around a person or a memory close to your heart can make the difference in how you feel on a daily basis. Focus on the emotion of love to synchronize your heart to a coherent rhythm. Another way to increase vital force is by hugging someone. Author Virginia Satir says, "We need four hugs a day for survival, eight hugs a day for maintenance, and twelve hugs a day for growth." If there is no one around to hug, hug a tree, an endless supply of energy. Realize that there is such as a thing as hug deficiency. Your intention to heal allows you to reverse stress and illness as soon as you decide. Disease becomes a choice, as does using your voice and opening your heart.

The alternative is to allow life to dictate your health. If the symptoms of dis-ease worsen over the years without relief, if you ignore what you put into your mouth, if you fail to speak your voice or close yourself off to receiving love, your body and soul will reach a tipping point. After years of self-neglect or self-flaggelation your body-soul will consult with your spirit and decide whether or not to take the path of least resistance to the next dimension. But up until that point, there are many opportunities to reverse or prevent further damage. There are many chances to awaken to the Self. Listen to all your bodies. If you believe life is a gift, choose the path of least resistance toward health. Take the whole body, mind, and spirit into account. To improve ourselves in this way allows us to become attuned to the direction of the spirit, our inner guidance.

Chapter Twelve

BUILDING BELIEFS

Y ou are powerful because the world you see is really a projection of how you see the world. Your thoughts and beliefs determine your life as it unfolds. You experience your life as *you* are, not as things are. As you believe, you think. As you think, you create.

We each begin to create our reality when we are born. We take our first breath, feel our first touch, taste our first drink, hear our mother's voice, and see the world around us. With each moment, our cells divide, grow, and are replaced by new cells. Each new cycle builds on previous experience. At the very core of our being we create whether we believe we are creators or not. We take the next breath.

Belief systems feed perceptions. Perceptions feed creativity. Creativity feeds experience. And experience creates reality. Therefore reality is merely a perception that goes back to a belief system.

Belief → thoughts and perceptions → creativity → reality

"Perception is reality."

~Lee Atwater, political strategist

Each person perceives reality differently because each person builds a unique belief system. The main tools used for building belief systems are: 1) cognitive resonance which opens the mind to new beliefs, and 2) cognitive dissonance that closes the mind to new beliefs. Beliefs are not good or bad. They don't make an individual better or worse, they merely make an individual reality. Whether the mind is open or closed depends upon the will of the ego.

Day by day, moment-by-moment we create an individual reality with each choice we make. And because we are all connected to each other in the morphic field we also create a collective realty. This collective reality stays in place as long as the collective consciousness supports and validates it. Today's world-view is a collective belief about life as it relates to science, medicine, religion, politics, economics, etc. and they all happen to be based in the educational system.

When we first began our schooling, our parents made the choice of school we would attend. They made the choice for us because they had more knowledge. And we were told to go to school to gain knowledge. However, we were too young to understand the difference between knowledge and knowing. If our belief on that first day of school was that we would share our unique gifts with the group, we soon learned that we would have to leave that belief at the door. In the classroom we were given new standards. We were told to sit still even if we wanted to dance, to form a line even if we wanted to make a circle. These standards would be our new measuring stick to see how well we matched up to the goals we had come to attain.

"The greatest obstacle to discovery is not ignorance it is the illusion of knowledge."

~Daniel J. Boostin, author "The Discoverers"

In receiving a free education, we accepted the illusion of knowledge which created obstacles to our creativity. We exchanged imagination and discovery for a belief system that was handed to us. In doing so, we neglected our true essence and denied our natural curiosity which became buried under rules and instructions to which we conformed. Over time, we put on rose-colored glasses that came as a free gift and everything old was new again. We forgot how to ask questions.

We became complacent. When life disappointed, we either laughed it off or used the mantra: "This is as good as it gets."

Today we are a nation in conflict living in a world in conflict where the field of science has become a wide-spread belief. Rupert Sheldrake, biologist and author of *Science Set Free: 10 Paths to New Discovery* says, "The science delusion is the belief system that science already understands the nature of reality in principle leaving any of the details to be filled in." [344]

Whereas science was once based on hypothesis, investigation, reason, analysis, and evidence, science today is conducted under a belief known as scientism that claims science alone renders truth about the world and reality. Today's science is based in materialism where everything is reduced to matter. Materialist science says that we are just our bodies, so that when the brain is dead, there is no consciousness and no life after death. All reductionist sciences have become "wholly-owned subsidiaries of this new world view." In his book, Sheldrake lays out ten dogmas of science then turns them into questions to see if they hold up to scrutiny.

Sheldrake proposes that several dogmas in society form the basis of our current educational system which are reinforced by systems of governments, medical research, and mainstream science. Some of the dogmas that underlie our systems include: 1) Nature is machine-like, 2) matter is unconscious, 3) Nature is purposeless, 4) the mind is inside your head, and 5) the laws of Nature are fixed. However, when this default world-view of science is questioned and all evidence is taken into account, dogmas begins to fall apart.

All self-organizing systems – atoms, molecules, cells, tissues, organs, organisms, and societies – are organized by morphic fields. At each level or peer group, morphic fields have intelligence and memory so that each system – crystals, plants, animals, humans – each have a collective memory of previous experience.

"...from top to bottom a plant is all leaf, united so inseparably with the future bud that one cannot be imagined without the other"

~Johann Wolfgang von Goethe, "Metamorphosis of Plants" 1906

Since morphic fields are defined by attractors (like attracts like), like-patterns tend to repeat. Once a new pattern takes shape, its field becomes stronger through repetition (as in Tiller's pH experiment). Through morphic resonance, patterns become more probable, more habit-forming, or instinct-forming as in animals. "The force that these fields exert is the force of habit," says Rupert Sheldrake.

This resonant force may explain why history tends to repeat itself even though we should know better. But knowing does not derive from knowledge. When people begin to yield to the curiosity of their inner child and question world-view beliefs of any system, awareness grows and perceptions change. As perceptions change, support for old paradigms naturally fall apart. Humanity can break any bad habit once we realize we have a responsibility to act on new truths. Only when we act do we witness the dismantling of false systems. In the case of scientism, the jig is up.

"Knowledge speaks but wisdom listens."

~Jimi Hendrix, musician, singer, songwriter

Graham Hancock, author, researcher, and speaker on supernatural phenomenon says, "Many scientists should admit that consciousness is the greatest mystery of science and that we don't know exactly how it works."[345] Hancock argues that altered states of consciousness, including dream states, have played a fundamental role in the evolution of human culture. At the same time, none of these altered states contradict or conflict with the conscious states that are valued by society – the problem solving and alert states.

When people perceive that a model is broken or hollow, when answers to questions do not line up, reality begins to turn. The answers are always found within each of us, just beneath the rose-colored glasses. The glasses are the filter that can limit or open awareness to new truths, thereby limiting or expanding our true potential. With the ego clogged with rules, opinions, and distractions it is no wonder we remain stuck in a dissonant paradigm. How do we regain our true power? Only when we remove the glasses will we be able to see the path we have traveled, refocus our vision, and make the choice to take a new path.

Duality Reality

In our ego-driven, divide-and-conquer world, we live in a duality reality. This reality reflects a matrix of opposites: introvert/extrovert, beginning/end, living/dead, mind/matter, wave/particle, self/other, material/spiritual, on/off, right/left. The hierarchical systems in which we find ourselves, from prisons to politics are grounded in duality, promoting separation over unity, creating leaders and followers. Our hierarchical system is served well by the Hegelian Dialectic.

The Hegelian Dialectic originated with George Hegel, a nineteenth century school teacher, who argued that human nature is a series of conflicts and resolutions that eventually elevate humankind to a unified spiritual state. The process is based in three easy steps: Problem-Reaction-Solution. Create a problem. Foment a reaction (of anger or sympathy). Provide a solution.[346]

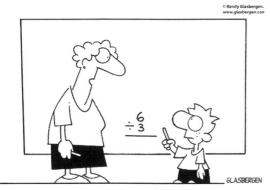

"No, we're just learning how to divide. When you get to business school, you'll learn how to divide and conquer."

Two hundred years later, whatever Hegel's good intentions, the goal to achieve unity from conflict-resolution has remained unproven and false. In duality reality, economic chaos has produced increased taxation. Shortages of oil and food have reinforced monopolies. The threat of pandemics has led to vaccine mandates. And the threat of terrorism has resulted in restrictions on individual freedoms. Conflict has only bred more conflict.

The obvious truth that refutes Hegel's idea is that unity is not uniformity. Unity follows no leaders and leads no followers. Unity does not restrict, limit, or conform through education or through more regulations and mandates. Unity is futile where players must choose to align with a tribe and plug into the implicit biases of tribal programming. The tribe – wearing the suits of political parties or the robes of religious sects – reinforces the divisions and the information that we already believe and want to hear.

Hegel's goal for unity cannot work because in duality reality we naturally choose competition over compassion. In our system of choosing sides
we lose our individuality. We hope for peace and wonder why nothing ever
changes. Those who believe they are on the side of peace accuse others of
being on the side of war. Each group fights with weapons of words, never
able to find peace, unity, or common ground because the very foundation of the system keeps people divided. Each side feels threatened by the
other in a struggle over control. The duality matrix creates winners and
losers. The media reinforces the infighting that keeps both sides distracted while an imbalance of power is maintained – the few controlling the
many. The many are promised protection and security against all their
fears. However, no guarantees are granted. As a consequence, the many
are left feeling vulnerable and powerless, embracing their servitude and
begging for greater protections at the expense of their freedoms.

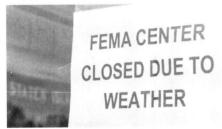 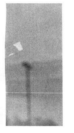

As a nation, we
experience the fear
of vulnerability every
time we are faced with
the consequences of
an unexpected natu-
ral, or man-made dis-
aster. We have become
dependent on the guise of security in the form of the National Weather
Service and the Federal Emergency Management Agency (FEMA) – so
much so that when the information is incorrect and the system fails, we
are left helpless, not knowing how to forage for food, build shelter, or fend
for ourselves as our ancestors did. We are a technically advanced nation
without a community and without a connection to the land on which we
live.

We believe that in giving our allegiance to the State and Federal
government that we are protected. However, the State, including local law enforcement has no duty to protect us. The Supreme Court
revealed this truth in 1856 in *South v. Maryland* when it ruled, "Local
law-enforcement had no duty to protect individuals but only a general
duty to enforce the laws.[347] The Supreme Court uses the Constitution
to protect the State in it's ruling in *Bowers v. Devito*: "there is no constitutional right to be protected by the state against being murdered
by criminals or madmen. The Constitution is a charter of negative

liberties; it tells the state to let the people alone; it does not require the federal government or the state to provide services, even so elementary a service as maintaining law and order."[348] There is no mutual obligation. In exchange for your vote to the system, you receive a false sense of security.

Our inherent rights do not come from the Constitution or the Bill of Rights, or any paper document. They are merely symbols. Inherent rights and freedoms are not dictated by regulations and statutes but by common sense and morals, as long as no harm or loss is caused. As endless wars throughout history have shown, it is futile to try to change a system from within a system. Author, philosopher and systems theorist, Richard Buckminster Fuller wrote, "You never change things by fighting the existing reality. To change something, build a new model that makes the existing model obsolete." For any system to change, core beliefs of those in the system must change.

Power vs. Force

Ending duality systems does not have to entail war. There is no true power in using force, as David R. Hawkins writes in his book, *Power vs. Force*. There is a big difference between power and force. Force always creates counterforce because it moves against opposition, whereas power is like gravity and moves within its field. Force is incomplete and needs energy whereas power is complete and makes no demands. Force consumes whereas power energizes. Power gives energy and life whereas force takes it away. Power is compassion whereas force is judgmental. Power is peace whereas force is war.[349]

The division of opposites will continue to play out in reality until we recognize that all war and peace, introvert and extrovert, light and dark exists within us. To attack another is to attack one's very nature. To judge another is to judge one's self.

We have chosen to create a separated consciousness but we can just as easily choose a one consciousness. We can opt out or withdraw consent from any system in peaceful resistance. Just saying no is powerful. Choosing not to participate in a system that doesn't serve the greatest good is making an energy statement as powerful as choosing to participate. Withdrawing consent is not apathy but the opposite of apathy. Knowing is power. Freedom is power. Standing in truth is power. Power is choosing kindness as your tribe. Fear of the unknown is the only power that holds us back. Once free of the system, you discover true liberty and the ability to know yourself and make decisions for yourself.

The truth is that there is never the need for a victor. There are no winners and losers in Oneness. The divisions we create are illusions from generations of conditioning. There is no need to choose the light side over the dark side, only to accept and transcend both sides to find wholeness. There is no need to choose a leader-ruler since the best leaders are equals. With such an awakening, there is no longer the need to prove one's self to others, only to love one's self and follow one's passion.

Spiritual author Eckhart Tolle writes about spiritual awakening as something meant to happen for the greater whole and its purpose. He describes this shift as the "disruption of outer purpose." Connection to one's dark side is necessary to bring about a deeper awareness to discovering one's inner purpose, after which the arising of a deeper outer purpose is aligned with the inner. By simply living our passions, we come to know our purpose. Both passion and purpose are found within. We all have our own truths and they all lead to the same place. As others discover these truths, the old Hegelian system will be seen for what it is, a hollow shell that eventually implodes from its own artificial weight.

A translation of Buddha's wisdom states: No one saves us from ourselves. No one can and no one may. We ourselves must walk the path.[350] No matter how often we blame the system, it is our collective core beliefs that have brought us to this point in time. The individual power struggle is mirrored in the power struggles of whole nations. The collective is reflected in the individual.

If you find yourself always coming up to the same unhappy, predictable outcome then might be time to reevaluate your internal wiring and change what you broadcast. If you find yourself feeling drained by your relationship with your partner or your friends, there is a strong chance that you also feel drained in other areas of your life. The symptoms of focusing on one area of life – your profession or relationship – do not bring about true balance. For that you must identify the cause. Go within. Take deep breaths. Listen for the answers. Stop resisting. Stand in your power. Make some changes.

Chapter Thirteen

CHANGING PARADIGMS

Today is your golden opportunity to make some changes and create a new paradigm. What better time than the present? First, you must shut down the logical brain and open the mind. Turn down the volume of the chatter in your head and open the heart. Listen to the messages around you and be aware of how they make you feel. Pay attention to the feelings that make you question what you are doing even if you have been doing it for as long as you can remember.

Be aware how many of our beliefs are fed to us daily. We easily believe what we hear and read without question, especially when repeated by those we admire. Consider the phrases, "natural health" and "alternative medicine." The truth is that health is, and always has been, our natural state, and likewise, alternative medicine has been our original medicine. We have embraced disease-based medicine as the standard measure of health even though disease is the absence of health. Using synthetic drugs to come to "wellness" for symptomatic relief is different from true "healing." Healing happens when we focus on cause rather than effect.

"Mental illness, of course, is not literally a 'thing'-or physical object- and hence it can 'exist' only in the same sort of way in which other theoretical concepts exist."

~Thomas Szasz, psychiatrist, social critic

Accepting a diagnosis of "mental illness" is taking on someone else's opinion based on belief and observation. However, dealing with the emotional cause (fear, anger, repression), heals the physical body. Changing thought patterns and belief systems realigns energy meridians to shift the state of physical organ systems.

Within a few generations, our two brains have become conditioned not to question the contradictions staring us in the face, and the gut. Today, "organic food" and "raw milk" are no longer simply "food" and "milk." Processed and nutritionally-dead foods are "new and improved," while live foods must be sterilized and irradiated before being allowed into the food supply. Tumors are treated with radiation and chemicals knowing that radiation and chemicals are proven carcinogens.[351] Mercury is regulated as a "hazardous waste in our external environment, but deemed "medically safe" for our internal environment in the form of vaccines and dental amalgams. We can overturn the conditioning that has molded our belief systems and limited our full potential by first being aware the conditioning exists.

In addition to being aware of language, pay attention to the feelings experienced in any given situation. If a spouse, or the tribe, claims you to be a threat to what they stand for, realize you have a choice in how you respond. You can take on their anger and let it drain you or you can let it go. You can choose not to become embroiled in an escalating argument if you don't make it personal. Instead of reacting with counterforce, step into your power and walk away. Breathe through any tightness. Realize that only those who lack self-confidence could ever feel threatened by another person's belief. They cannot be controlled by the thoughts of another person unless they allow it.

Words of attack are often a projection from the sender based in fear rather than a reflection of the receiver. Instead of taking on other people's opinions of who you are, start believing in your own essence. Other people's opinions about your character are none of your business because others see from their own perspective. You can never please those who do not want to be pleased. You cannot make them happy just as you do not make them angry. Each person creates these emotions from within. Separate yourself from the chaos. Release the tightness. Keep your energy and leave them theirs.

Intuitive Children

As adults, our beliefs have shaped our limited ways of thinking and prevented us from seeing the bigger picture. Our children are the ones who will lead us to a new level of awareness and existence. We can learn by their examples, their openness, and their compassion. But we have to be able to hear with open minds and hearts. Children are intelligent and need much more stimulation than they receive. We cannot teach them in the ways in which we were raised but in the ways they deserve to be raised or they will quickly unlearn the pure knowledge they bring.

In the words they choose they offer insight, as when a young boy of ten told his mother that he has always been with her, always been a part of her, even before she was born as part of the egg from which she was formed.[352] Such wisdom from the mouth of babes resonates in truth. It makes intuitive sense. They understand the nature of nonlocality – the theory of relativity as consciousness – without ever having taken a physics class. Their connection to the collective consciousness is strong.

> *"From a very early age, I've had to interrupt my education to go to school."*
>
> *~George Bernard Shaw*

Sadly, our school systems are not equipped for the children that are here now, let alone for the ones who are coming. Universal schooling suffers from the same malady as universal medicine. It is not intuitive to treat everyone the same when each is unique. Many children in today's educational system are seen as problems – as square pegs in round holes. They are labeled Attention Deficit, and medicated to control behavior to a standardized uniformity. Children become deadened to what is happening around

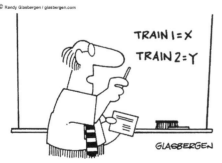

© Randy Glasbergen / glasbergen.com

TRAIN 1 = X
TRAIN 2 = Y

GLASBERGEN

"If Train #1 leaves Los Angeles at 8:47 AM going 63 MPH and Train #2 leaves New York at 9:13 AM going 56 MPH, how long will it take for your mind to wander to something more interesting?"

them and that affects their ability to think clearly, to be creative, and think for themselves. The dumbing-down process evident in our educational system produces children who lose their sense of Self.

Overmedication creates imbalances at the level of the cell membrane, and interferes with children's innate connection to their natural environment. The aura is also affected, making kids vulnerable to energy leaks and blocking them from full vitality.

Without the "chemical lobotomy" of mind-altering drugs, today's children are acutely aware and clairvoyant because they work from the heart.[353] They are so strongly self-aware because of their connection with universal laws that they will resist the confinement of the current school system where everyone is lumped together and made to conform through rote learning. Children who suppress their gifts do so from fear of being different. This creates a disconnection with the physical body, which leads to behavioral and health problems. Since our children are more open than ever, they also understand more than we can appreciate. They will create the new paradigm.

Learn, Unlearn and Relearn

American writer and futurist Alvin Toffler wrote, "The illiterate of the 21st century will not be those who cannot read and write, but those who cannot learn, unlearn, and relearn." Today, schooling must adapt from a rigid education structure to an open, emotion-based place of learning. It must take the whole person into account versus classifying individuals based solely on academic achievement. The focus needs to be experimentation over repetition, creativity over competition, innovation over memorization, and freedom and flexibility over abuse of authority. We must create a space in which the teacher is an equal learning companion, where energy flows in both directions, as in the model of harmonic resonance.

Current learning is focused on the thinking brain (prefrontal cortex), but life happens in other regions of the brain (temporal lobe, the brain steam, spinal cord, cerebellum, sacrum etc.,) and throughout the body based on stimuli from our environment. Every time you learn something new your brain physically changes.[354] Therefore, what is learned in school must be applicable to daily life. Children need to experience a sense of cultural identity in a global world, a place with a sense of purpose. Schools must change with and for the children because it will be the children born today who lead us to a healthier paradigm. Schools already exist where there is no bullying or violence or substance abuse, or stress. The Waldorf Schools "play to learn" vs. learn to play. In other schools children meditate ten minutes twice a day. Young children do walking meditation. They release stress. They stop fidgeting. Free play and meditation allow kids to consolidate skills just learned. They use their whole brain and connect to their higher selves to find clarity to open to their creativity. The benefits are many in schools around the world where meditation (not medication) is practiced.[355]

The Leap of Faith

Changing paradigms means that when you feel you are suddenly in the spotlight of your life, having to make a decision to maintain the status quo or take a leap of faith, simply allow your gut feeling to guide you. Your gut resides in the third chakra, the solar plexus, the house of your personal power. Don't fear your power even when it does not come with statistics, charts, grids, or representatives. If the third chakra is weak or stuck, then you lack confidence and self-esteem. You feel uncomfortable in different situations. You experience digestive disorders. When balanced and moving, your third chakra allows you to express your power easily. Instead of life getting you down, you experience life propping you up.

If you take a leap of faith, hold no investment in the outcome. This is the definition of letting go. When you don't create expectations, chances are you won't be disappointed. Put on your no-fear dancing shoes and take the first awkward step. Don't be afraid to stumble. Oscar Wilde, one of the most successful English playwrights of his day, said, "Experience is the name we give to our mistakes." Simply be open to the possibilities, bruises and all.

"We make mistakes and mistakes make us."

~Anthony Douglas Williams, "Inside the Divine Pattern"

After all, life is a series of first-hand experiences. And experience is the result of one's thoughts *and* actions. Monitor your own stream of consciousness so you can identify negative thoughts to change belief patterns that need to shift. People often say they want things to change but they also admit they don't like change at all because it is never what they expect. They are conflicted within themselves so they end up sending mixed signals that result in self-sabotage. As the artist of your life's masterpiece – you must attempt to paint. You cannot just dream about it. There is a big difference between setting an intention and taking action. Know what you want to do then go out and do it.

For anything to change, you must be open and willing to change. When beliefs and thoughts shift, awareness shifts. When you can see your past mistakes without regret, you see with new eyes. In coming "full circle," your axis shifts and rocks your world.

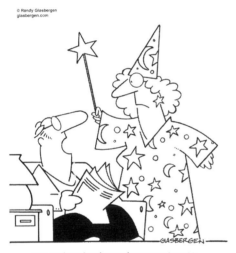

"Remember what the marriage counselor said? It only works if I <u>want</u> to change!"

When shift happens, it is natural to want to share your new vision and enthusiasm with those closest to you. You may take on new philosophies about food and begin to cook differently. Your political or religious views might shift one hundred eighty degrees. You might stop watching TV. Your choices reverberate to affect those around you, causing ripples and eddies. Expecting others to fall in line builds resistance. Others cannot be forced to join you in your new spiritual growth orbit. Pushing them to see things your way when they are not ready will only serve to push them away. Achieving control over others is an illusion. Many times, women attempt to do too much in relationships with both family and men. Always doing for others means women don't trust others to be strong enough to make their own choices for their own growth.

On a deeper level, making others happy at one's own expense may reflect a lack of self-love, stemming from a deep fear of loss. The loss is something that may have happened long ago, perhaps lifetimes ago, and keeps coming up. Emotional loss, weakness, or feelings of instability are commonalities we refuse to acknowledge within ourselves. In all relationships there is an energy exchange. Each person gets something out of it. Staying in an abusive relationship happens because the one suffering abuse receives a certain security in familiar pain. The abused person gives over power to the abuser to fill a perceived need. In relationships where a couple assumes a parent-child dynamic, the one who needs to be coddled will also put up with orders and demands from the other who needs to assert control. They set each other up.

Instead of blaming our emotions on a situation or another person, we need to face up to a deficiency of power from within, and fulfill it from there. Our feminine side (yin) must reach up to merge with our masculine side (yang) to reach wholeness. The merging of yin and yang happens through the heart. Focus your attention there. If a void exists it is because you have most likely given your power away.

Fortunately, it is not too late to reverse the condition. Visualize the void of the heart fill with the light of love and this time create an expandable, porous container that allows this energy to flow in all directions. Love knows no bounds or limits, though it must be nourished. Allow the light to fill the container and watch the container expand. The size of the container is only limited by your imagination. See the edges of the light flame up to incinerate old patterns, programs, beliefs, doubts, fears, anything you want to release. You have everything you need. You have the strength to dissolve relationships that no longer serve you. You can attract others who are also filled with love. In a world where all things are possible each of us unfolds into our own potential. So too, will society unfold.

> *"You have your way, I have my way. As for the right way, the correct way, the only way, it does not exist."*
>
> *~Friedrich Nietzsche*

In navigating relationships, we need to appreciate that people paint the world how they see it. You may have painted *life under the microscope* but the other person sees *life under the night sky*. You're each seeing from a different place. Accept the fact that both of your perceptions are valid. You are a unique creative force surrounded by other unique creative forces. You always have a choice about what you create and how you create it. Everyone's truth is unique. There is no one right answer so why fight about it? If change is necessary, don't wait for the other person. Allow change for yourself. Trust yourself. If there is ever a right way, it is the way of *your* truth.

When it comes to making life changes, you can either languish in the status quo, ever comforted by complacency, trying to live up to others' expectations, or you can embark on a journey of your own choosing. You can decide to accept another's truth for yourself or discover that you might have your own. In this dimension there are universal truths that shape the greater reality. But there is also your truth, unique to you and your world. Whatever it is you want to change, think it, feel it, then grab it with both hands.

Unleash Your Inner Child

If your adult self continues to resist inevitable change, it might be time to unleash the child within. Your inner child has always been there as you've grown up. Your child sees the world with enthusiasm, joy, and curiosity. Imagination rules. Adventure reigns. Dreams are actualized. Each day is truly a new world with unknown opportunities. Everything is fresh. The child looks for ways to feed the imagination using all the senses. You sense your way from one experience to another based on what feels good. You absorb them. You have a blind spot to obstacles because self-expression of your creativity is the first priority. This child is your spirit that makes space for you to create with all the tools of your vast imagination. She circulates the creative juices in movement and dance. He marvels in the sound from a blade of grass and the blue of the sky.

Do you still recognize this child or have time, responsibilities, and obligations pushed aside curiosity and awe? It's likely you hardly noticed the change. Insidiously, the shadows of uncertainty, frustration, and fear took hold merely because your perceptions changed. You began to compare yourself to others and make excuses for the lost child when priorities changed. Inspiration faded. Creativity took a backseat to duties. Action turned to inaction or reaction. You escaped into the pages of a novel, a trip to the mall, or your work. Negativity moved in and decided to stay.

Just because the child grew into larger shoes does not mean he or she is not still there waiting patiently to be noticed. He might just reintroduce you to that old paintbrush sitting in the box behind the stairs. She may drag you out on the dance floor and remind you how you used to do that thing with your hips. Go for a run. Hide out in the woods. Climb a tree. Play chess. Take up karate. Anything is possible when you allow your inner child to take you gently by the hand and lead you into the unknown.

Chapter Fourteen

LAW OF ATTRACTION

You attract what you focus on with amazing accuracy. This is reflected in the universal Law of Attraction. Thought energy you generate, positive or negative, will direct your cells to vibrate at that frequency. Self-worth, self-doubt, self-love all become bodily responses based on your beliefs. Like attracts like. If you doubt this, try it out for yourself.

If you are ready to enter into a new relationship but you keep coming up empty, listen to what you tell yourself and what you tell others. When you talk to yourself in silence, you are also listening. Is your stream of consciousness a contradiction of thoughts?

Do you say, "I want someone in my life but I can't seem to attract a partner?" Do you tell others, "They always say that I'm funny and smart and fun to be with but they don't seem to find me attractive. They should take a chance on me, but in reality, most people are either too hurt to think about a relationship or they're just not interested. I've really given up on it. I'm comfortable with my singlehood. I don't need a partner in my life to be a whole person."

Three words: Law of Attraction.

In another case, you may find yourself always feeling anxious when it comes to money because there is never enough to pay the bills. The anxious feeling lingers and keeps you awake at night so you have less energy during the day. You take our your frustration on your loved ones because misery enjoys company and because you need their positive energy just to maintain balance. The energy deficit you create in the household is manifested in the bank account. Feeling anxious without money creates more of the same. Why would you believe feeling positive would change anything financially since you've never seen it happen before in your experience?

Law of Attraction.

The universe does not judge, even if you do. It merely gives you more of what you are. Like your very DNA, you are a beacon, a sender and receiver of information. Therefore, how you think, what you think, and more importantly how you feel becomes critical to your well-being and your results. Being clear as mud will get you a dirty floor. That is why taking time to breathe and writing down the thoughts that muddle your mind helps you separate what you don't want from what you do want.

> *"Whatever the present moment contains, accept it as if you had chosen it."*
>
> *~Eckhart Tolle, spiritual author*

For instance, if you want someone to come into your life, you should not say the words, "I want someone in my life," and then cancel it by saying how comfortable you are with being single. Instead, create a list of all the qualities you desire in a mate, a sort of no-holds-barred blueprint. Create space in your life by clearing out a closet. Then embody the feeling of seeing your blueprint come to life. Next, create a list of the things you love about yourself. Write at least twenty-five qualities. Dig deep. Go over the list daily until they roll off the tongue. You know who you are.

If you want the money to flow to you, then begin to feel that you already have enough. Find your attractor field, that feeling of being complete and satisfied, even if it means splurging on a spa weekend with lots of back rubs and flowing water. Understand that money is simply a form of energy and you are the catalyst for its transformation. Fully relax in the realization that each drop of water represents real value into your hands, since it does. And remember that water has memory too. During the time you have shifted your thoughts, your cells have shifted their own vibration. Continue this feeling whenever you hear water. Shower often.

There doesn't have to be any shortages in water, food, money, or love. It all flows to you from that place deep within your own well. You only have to believe it and retrieve it. At the same time, notice those around you. The people closest to you reflect back who you are at the core. They often echo your thoughts in their words. Anything that bothers you is reflective of work needing to be done on yourself. No matter who they are, what they say, or how they may have behaved, they are all gifts to appreciate. They have helped bring you to this moment of self-awareness.

Three words: You are loved.

Fear cannot exist inside of love. Others who have come and gone are not evil or good. They are a reference point for everything going on inside of us. They show us the cause of our symptoms. And in many cases, the cause is based in our undigested emotions – the fear of intimacy, the fear of getting hurt again, the fear of change, or the fear of standing in our own power. If you cannot hear the wisdom of your own words, listen closely to those nearest you. If you want to see love, be love. The challenge is to awaken to the fear that is stopping you.

Go Down to the Well

Everyone faces challenges. You can always choose to resist change or go where the flow takes you. You always have a choice. Even if you don't know where you are going, take a chance and get wet. Begin to feel the emotions you have buried or they will keep bubbling up. Question from where these emotions come. If you are crying for no apparent reason, let the tears fall anyway. Then wipe them away. Rinse and repeat as often as necessary. Be patient with yourself. The purpose is not to stay dry even if that towel wrapped around you is more comfortable. Be ready to unwrap your emotions and bear your soul. There is no harm in getting completely wet. Just as you earlier took that leap of faith, now take the plunge. Come into your power. The water will be the right temperature. You only have to surrender to it. Allow the current of fear to flow through you. As you release the block, new energy will flow in bringing with it what you choose. The only one holding you back is you.

"Each morning when I open my eyes I say to myself: I, not events, have the power to make me happy or unhappy today. I can choose which it shall be. Yesterday is dead, tomorrow hasn't arrived yet. I have just one day, today, and I'm going to be happy in it.

~Groucho Marx, comedian

There are plenty of sources of artificial fear being broadcast in our collective biofield that reinforce the fears we feel, the media being the most obvious. But you can choose not to receive that broadcast and not to rebroadcast to others. Turn off the TV, cancel the newspaper subscription, choose your Facebook friends wisely, and make it your intention to filter out negative thoughts. You are in control. By changing your reception you change your broadcast.

Remember, your beliefs and perceptions alter your biology at every moment in time. By adjusting your perceptions and assumptions, you rewrite your very genes. You change your behavior. If your behavior doesn't change then you truly have not changed your assumptions. The outcomes of your life come from you.

See Yourself as You Are

Choose to see yourself as your spirit sees you, as ageless. You are not getting older. You are as young as you feel. Your biological Earth age is not reflective of your mind age or your spirit age. You are a being of at least three different timelines. As an Earth being, you are newly born each day as your cells continuously remake themselves. As a soul being, you are ageless and infinite since time and space do not exist outside of this dimension. As a mind being, you are wise beyond your Earth years because you choose not to accept labels about age. Be open to all the possibilities. Believe forty-eight is the new twenty-eight. Whether it is a question of age or health or love, when you are open to new ideas, you make an energy statement. You literally change your vibration, your cells, and your potential.

"As you think so shall you become."

~Bruce Lee, martial artist

When you raise your thoughts and emotions to the positive, you take control of your life from the inside out. It is important to appreciate the uniqueness that is you no matter your age or your perceived flaws. The definition of flaw is a mark, fault, or other imperfection. If you stand back and use your artist eye to blur your vision, notice that "imperfect" is really "I'm perfect." Understand that the meaning of "appreciate" is to "increase in value." Each time you take time to appreciate yourself and those around you, you increase their value for yourself and for the world. You shift your vibration to align with your highest potential and in doing so you send a ripple of your energy out to the rest of world. It is your truth emanating. Truth is always simple. Align with your true nature. Don't get caught up in the labels of good or bad, right and wrong. There is no good or bad. There only perception.

Consciousness Rising

Nothing is static. The only constant is change. Even judgment evolves as we gain new insights. We have the choice of how we see things. We can choose to believe that there is no judgment in the vastness of the universe, only energy, shape-shifting from one form to another as we express our individuality.

Human consciousness shifts within its own morphic field just like all self-organizing systems. It learns from past experience, innovates, and moves itself forward, always seeking to know more. Divine consciousness lives in divine light. It does not live in duality. There is no center or left or right, or wrong. There is only infinite possibility and Oneness. We can promote extremes and opposition or we can choose to be neutral and integrate. The choice is for each of us to make on our own path.

When we are ready to stop reacting, we become open to allowing. When we shut down our rigid, programmed beliefs and preconceived ideas, old laws and whole systems – including systems that hold us in servitude – become obsolete. When we change the stories in our heads we change our outcomes. When we stop following the crowd, we stop "group think" to come into our own uniqueness. We expand consciousness from the five-sense body-mind level to include all our senses, to feel and to know that we all come from one infinite consciousness.

In rewriting our perception or judgment or any emotion, we rewrite our collective story on all levels. We remove the filter of the ego and open our minds. Our ability to change anything in the collective human experience is based on each of us as individuals being willing to part ways with the past. The process is a personal one. There is no need to push or attack or judge anyone else's process. When our frequency changes we draw new people and experiences that resonate in our new way of believing, thinking, and being. In the process, people leave, jobs change, and attitudes change. Like an echo, what we send out comes back. When our sense of perception changes, our sense of personal power shifts. All of reality evolves. We free ourselves. We come into harmony with our higher intelligence. We pull ourselves up into that spiral. We come together. We heal.

THE SPIRIT

Chapter Fifteen

RECONNECTING TO SPIRIT

*"It is time to speak your truth.
Create your community,
Be good to each other.
Do not look outside yourself for a leader.*

*There is a river flowing now very fast.
It is so great and swift
That there are those who will be afraid.
They will try to hold onto the shore.
They will feel they are being pulled apart
And will suffer greatly.*

*Understand that the river knows its destination.
The elders say we must let go of the shore,
Push off into the middle of the river,
Keep our eyes open and our heads above water."*

~The Elders, Oraibi, Arizona Hopi Nation

The nature of healing happens on multiple levels and in many layers. It is a process of disrobing and being comfortable in your own skin. True healing is the ability to stand in naked truth and feel free to fully express yourself.

In expressing our filled up selves, we must be willing to suspend disbelief. We must see ourselves beyond the mirror as one body-mind-spirit being. As spirit beings, we come directly from Source energy. We are formless, dimensionless, pure light energy, ever-expanding, spiraling outward. We are the stuff of the universe in its basic elements. We bring life.

In order to grow in awareness and in love, spirit beings split into individual soul beings, similar to how a cell divides. The soul body holds the essence of spirit that is the spark of Source known as the higher self. The higher self is the wise, calm aspect of the soul that enjoys an expanded awareness through access to higher realms and guidance. We find the higher self during states of meditative silence and in stillness. As individual soul bodies, we are not only able to access this higher, enlightened state of creativity, but our light energy is also able to compact itself to form molecules and become dense enough to form the physical body.

We are more than meets the eye. We are also beings of many subtle bodies. The most commonly known energy bodies are the etheric-body, the astral-body, the memory (causal) body, the emotional, the mental body, and the soul-body. The etheric body blends the physical and the etherial dimensions. It is of the same size and shape as the physical body and surrounds every cell, and thereby transfers life force into each cell. The memory body contains past experiences and patterns. The mental body is also known as the intuitive body. The emotional-body is the body of desires and emotions, imagination, and psychic abilities. The astral body allows one to travel to the dream world during sleep. It is the portal for visions, hallucinations, and out of the body/near death experiences. The soul-body interpenetrates both physical and etheric bodies, and when developed, acquires the ability to perceive the *inner world* (clairvoyance, etc.). Beyond these subtle bodies lies the life force, the current of light and sound from where healing ability stems.[356]

All subtle bodies are specific fields of electromagnetic energy layered on top of each other outside the physical body. Each body exists on its own plane. The mental body on the mental plane, the astral body on the astral plane, and so on. When the chakras are not aligned, flow is restricted and problems arise. Together these bodies form the aura that is perceptible to some people and can be photographed using Kirlian photography. Whereas the aura is more an energy that surrounds and reflects the metabolic processes of the physical body, the subtle bodies are thought to act as filters for teachings from the soul and higher self. They regulate the soul's activity on the physical plane.[357] It is as beings of both matter and light energy, that we experience our physical world.

"The spirit is life. The mind is the builder. The physical is the result."

~Edgar Cayce, American psychic

As a soul, you give life to the temple that is your body so that you can experience life through the physical senses (taste, touch, see, smell, and sound) as well as through the ethereal senses. Everything is connected. Your subtle bodies are connected to the physical body through various organs and glands. The etheric body is intertwined with the physical. The emotional body connects through the stomach, the astral body through the kidneys, the soul body through the pineal gland, and the integrated spiritual body through the pituitary. The right brain balances all of these bodies. In true health, the chakras of all subtle bodies are aligned and work in harmony with each other. Disease results when blockages occur or vibration among these bodies comes out of alignment.[358]

Though somewhat limited by our physical bodies, we are also forces of will and awareness and love. As the physical body is created for a finite time, our spirit is ageless and deathless. As infinite beings, we more than the notes in the musical scale and the colors of light spectrum. We are also everything in between.

Like fingers connected to a hand, we are here as an expression of the whole, to learn and grow and create, all influencing each other, all in communication with each other. The soul created the body to express itself in order to know itself. In claiming our bodies, we may have temporarily forgotten the essence of who we really are, and the Source from which we really came. But all is not lost. No one is lost or forgotten even as we face perceived hardship and suffering. The experience of a lifetime is purposeful in understanding polarity and duality. Like the transformation of a caterpillar to a butterfly, we are each under-going a metamorphosis to bring light and dark into balance so we are healed and transformed.

Since ultra-dimensional is who we are, we are built to live in two separate worlds: the physical and the spiritual. We are participants within our three-dimensional reality and also outside of it, here to mature both physically and spiritually. Universal laws govern the de-velopment of spiritual organs just as the laws of Nature and reason govern the development of the physical organs and the mind. Both are intertwined. If soul and mind are reflected in the physical body then a healthy spiritual disposition mirrors a healthy physical disposition.

As our physical selves evolve we see that we are connected to a higher self which is connected to a unified whole. We come to real-ize that the separateness we experience in our 3D time and space dimension is just an illusion. Nothing is as it seems. Einstein said that time – past, present, and future – is all happening at once. Everything is happening now. We exist in many dimensions simultaneously with multiple possibilities that arise each moment.

Since your soul essence is that part of you that is multidimension-al, you are spread out through an infinite range of possibilities. You have simultaneous selves – doppelgangers – who live out the path you could have taken. They live their own lives thinking they are the real you. The only difference between you in this dimension and you in other dimensions is where your awareness is focused, and in your abil-ity to shift between dimensions. Of course there could be another you who can shift frequencies as easily, and it might be instructive to be able to speak to a future you when making a decision to see how your choices might play out in this reality. Anything is possible when time is not an issue. Your essence is not any one physical self since the soul (consciousness) is multidimensional, spread out over a range of pos-sibilities. Shifting your consciousness to elsewhere is not dependent on what you are physically able to do here as you personally experience when you find yourself driving on autopilot, not knowing how you got from point a to point b. On your spiritual journey it is your responsibil-ity to discover the possibilities.

According to physicists Karl Pribram and David Bohm in their Holographic model of the universe, we are riding a wave of unlimited possibility in a Field from which everything is created. This soup of subatomic waves is projected from a dimension beyond our own that ripples outside both time and space to create reality.[359]

"We do not grow absolutely, chronologically. We grow sometimes in one dimension, and not in another, unevenly. We grow partially. We are relative. We are mature in one realm, childish in another. The past, present, and future mingle and pull us backward, forward, of fix us in the present. We are made of layers, cells, constellations."

~The Diary of Anaïs Nin Vol. 4 (1971); Journal of Phenomenological Psychology Vol. 15 (1984)

Professor John Hagelin, professor at Maharishi University says, "at the core of the universe is a single unified Field of intelligence that unites all the forces and particles of Nature that is the basis of everything, mind and matter."[360] This non-material Field describes matter as waves of vibration, a place where everything already exists, ideas conceived and those not yet conceived. And all of it exists in waveform. We live in what many believe to be a conceptual or "thought universe," acting out our lives on the stage of potential." Haglein believes the deeper we go, the less dense and the more conscious the universe becomes until there is only pure intelligence.

The Field or Hologram is the model that explains why memories are not only stored in the brain but throughout the body. It explains the inexplicable phenomenon of telepathy, precognition, and the paranormal. When we consider the vast possibilities that exist beyond what we see, we begin to appreciate our life and its capacity for the profound. Understanding that the physical universe is not so solid, but a malleable Field of potentiality that we create as we go, we become aware that we are all-powerful spiritual beings. We decide.

Accepting our spirituality means that amidst the physical chaos, there can be peace. In place of physical suffering, there can be happiness. All pain – emotional, physical, mental – is a symptom with a message. To ignore it or suppress it is to continue the suffering. All suffering comes from the idea of being separate from Source, from Self. The First Nobel Truth of Buddhism teaches: Pain is inevitable.

Suffering is optional. While there is suffering in life, Buddhism teaches that suffering comes from not getting what we want. It is a result of craving and clinging and prevents true happiness which is found within.

Suffering is ultimately a choice. Once we understand and accept pain's message, the pain goes away. Not everyone will find meaning or truth in this ancient teaching, but true spiritual teachers are careful to qualify that truth does not come from a person or enlightened being, but flows through them. Truth may come through tone, through rhythm or movement of body language, or through the words themselves. You know truth by the way it feels. The effect on one who hears or experiences truth is felt to the core. As a student of life, this is important to consider since finding your truth is part of the journey.

Life's journey may not always go the way you intend it to go. At times, it may be messy, sticky, and in need of a good housecleaning. We can become entangled in the contrasts around us where nothing makes sense. We may reach a point where we question everything we've ever been taught. Marcus Aurelius, philosopher and Roman emperor from 161 to 180 AD, wrote (as translated) "If you are troubled by external circumstances, it is not the circumstances that trouble you, but your own perception of them and they are within your power to change at any time."[361]

This spiritual emperor saw that everything comes from Nature and advocated for each of us find our place within the universe. Each circumstance is an opportunity for growth. Each experience is part of a plan to learn who we really are. In the process we peel away the layers that constrict. We gain access to our inner Self. We discover freedom from the limitations of the mind. We separate truth from opinion. We unlearn what we've been taught. We find balance in body, mind, and spirit. We come out of balance. We are always reacting to shifting energies even though we may not perceive it. To deny this cosmic part of ourselves is to deny who we really are.

Spirituality is your connection to your spirit, which is connected to everything. It is about being a servant of the planet and of humanity. This sense of connection helps in all aspects of life. When you have meaning and purpose in life you are not held captive by the contrasts around you. You don't see a reason to act your age because you understand that the soul is ageless. You are not trapped by fear because fear is only a perception. Before long you begin directing your life instead of reacting to it. Of course, spirituality has a practical application, too. As you gain a sense of fulfillment and self-satisfaction in life, you recover faster from disease, you are healthier in mind and body, and that gives rise to a longer life in good health.

"Spirituality is not about following, adoring, worshiping, or fearing. It does not judge. It does not restrict. It is always expanding, embracing, kind, nurturing, flexible, understanding, open, and loving. It is all about freedom not restraint. It is definitely not about convincing or converting others. It is all about empowering the Self which benefits all. Be free. Let your Spirits soar."

~Eric Allen, "The New Awakening"

Soul Family

We come here eager to learn. We put on a uniform, go to school, take off the uniform and eventually go home. While we are here, we work and we play. We love and we hate. Our classmates – our family, friends, and everyone we meet in life – make up our soul family. With them we experience the greatest accomplishments and the greatest struggles. We have more than one soul mate.

Like our human family, our soul family members are the people with whom we get along and those with whom we do not. They are lifelong friends and people who drift into our lives for a brief but intense, stay. They are whole communities that come in to assist each other. Our soul family is a group of acquaintances and those with whom we share a deep love and a spiritual bond that sets them apart from the superficial people in our lives. In his book, *The Journey of Souls*, Michael Newton's research shows that we experience many lifetimes and experiences with soul groups.[362] These are the ones who help us grow, evolve, and create spiritually, the ones who are very similar in frequency makeup.

Not only do we plan to rendez-vous with members of our soul family while in uniform, but we also write the main events that happen in our lives through soul contracts. In her book, *Sacred Contracts*, Medical Intuitive Caroline Myss writes that sacred contracts in human relationships can bring people together for reasons of romantic love but also for issues and problems beyond love relationships. We draw to others for personal growth but also for the greater good and for spiritual transformation. Conversations with these people are generally deep, personal, and about world issues.

Some souls we meet radiate qualities that are deeply attractive beyond the physical. When they are not around, we miss them. We might call these heart connections. This longing or ache can sometimes overpower us if we are not grounded. We can obsess about an emptiness we feel when not in their presence. This perceived deficiency or lack is a natural aspect of the physical body's need to attach itself to others. The key, again, is to recognize that while they may have sparked this emotion, the emptiness we feel has little to do with the other person. While they may indeed be a natural heart match, these souls are gifts who teach us that we still need to work to heal something in ourselves or the lesson will be repeated.

The need to be fulfilled by others is really reflective of the need to spiritually connect to the source of who we are. The light so attractive in others is really a reflection of our own light, the light of the cosmos. And no light is brighter or deeper. By grounding ourselves in this knowledge, we reconnect to our inner glow and we stop floating. We come out of the head that tells us we are empty and move into the heart that shows us we are full. The fog clears and we see with clarity. We reconnect to the love that is already here. We fill our cups without feeling the need to be filled up by others. Whether we are ready or not, we attract who we are.

The old idea of a soul mate as a romantic partner does not go far enough to capture the full complexity of heart connection. Heart connections are those we are bound to meet one way or another. No matter how many missed opportunities have passed us by, we eventually find each other through that universal Law of Attraction. Simply put, our frequencies oscillate in harmony with others who are like us. This is expressed through the concept of harmonic resonance.

Harmonic resonance is electromagnetic, a phenomenon in Nature that transcends physical matter. It is visually depicted as ripples that are generated when two similar stones are dropped in water at the same time and from the same height. When the waves of the stones are in sync, they converge on each other, overlap, and the combined power of the interacting waves is doubled. Harmonic resonance is seen in the luminosity of a sprinkle of fireflies. It is heard in the chirping of an orchestra of crickets. Each individual firefly or cricket will flash or chirp its own tune when kept in isolation but will synchronize with thousands of others when together out in the open.

As reflected in our closest soul family interactions, at the core of any successful harmonic relationship there is friendship. Without resonance there is dissonance or destructive interference. Energies that are out of sync cancel each other. Real friendship with a soul mate of the heart is love – pure, authentic, and sacred. No physical strings need be attached. When we find those who resonate with us in mind and heart, it may seem accidental. However, there are no accidents or co-incidences in Nature. We have come together – in harmony – through frequency matching, using echo location, much like our furry-winged, warm-blooded, milk-producing, flying counterpart, the bat. When we find our soul peeps it is meant to be. We find familiarity. Such a match can also be gleaned through numerology.[363]

Twin Souls

Of all soul reunions, the twin flame or twin soul reunion is thought to be the most fulfilling on all levels because it is believed to be magical and one of great intensity. Twin souls recognize each other on the level of the soul, through the sound of the voice or a feeling of familiarity, and not necessarily consciously.

The twin reunion can happen on any soul age level with complications depending on the maturity level of the soul.[364] Older souls tend to face complications due to life plan. They can be out of sync by age, peer group, locale, or lifestyle even though they can still meet physically and connect spiritually. Younger souls are more easily provoked into creating turmoil for themselves, but the connection is just as intense. Twin souls see themselves reflected in the eyes of the other. They feel as if they've always known each other. They feel like home. The evolution of twin souls begins after they split from one soul light body and condense to separate forms. Each soul presence is an electronic blueprint or an exact duplicate copy of the other. The masculine is electric, or active, and the feminine is magnetic, or attractive.

The story of twins is reflective of an unwinding spiral of a DNA molecule where the two souls go their separate ways, incarnating over and over – gathering human experience, practicing with others, learning about love, balancing male and female aspects, working together in the service of others – with the task of aligning with their spiritual and personal strengths. It is thought that each of us has only one twin and each twin is a complete soul. Both are aware of themselves as individuals, but also as one that is a being larger and more powerful than they are as individuals. The one who carries the divine feminine energy will magnetize or attract the one who carries the divine masculine energy. Eventually, twins will unite on all levels – physically, sexually, emotionally, and spiritually – fully merging to create the one energy. With this intense soul union, there is no baggage to weigh on the relationship. Healing on all levels will have taken place since both partners must be powerful and balanced within themselves.[365] This bond is unlike any other. It is not about one type of love. It is about love in all its forms.

If this evolution of souls appears to be a fairy tale of unlimited proportions then you have found your inner child. Congratulations. You will appreciate the ending. For when twins finally join as two complete and whole human beings it is said to be the ultimate relationship. Unlike a typical fairy tale, there is no ending. The soul growth and creativity experienced in this plane evolves to another. The love story continues. Quite a romantic notion to consider. With this knowledge, we are reassured that we are never alone. Love is always with us, found inside us, and mirrored in our twin, who will reunite with us eventually on the healing journey. Knowing we have a twin, we can fully immerse ourselves in all our relationships in order to work on ourselves. We can avoid conflict knowing that peace comes from transcending self-doubt. We can celebrate life knowing that our final twin reunion will be one to remember!

Many of us have purposefully chosen to forget our ethereal soul contracts after we arrive here. Yet many are now also seeking and accessing this information from what is known as the Akashic. The Aksahic is a word from ancient Sanskrit which means "Record." The Akashic records every event that has ever occurred within this universe. This history is written in the non-physical plane. Human beings have been interacting consciously and unconsciously with these records throughout history, both deliberately and accidentally, through insight and through dreams. The information of the Akashic is available everywhere and to everyone. Space and time do not affect the records, as this 'inner world' is non-local (without bounds) and ultra-dimensional.

The Record, however, does not record the lives of individuals. The lives of individuals are recorded in the brain (short-term memory) and in our DNA (long-term memory). In his book, *Synthesis*, Chris Thomas writes, "If we go to someone who can read past lives, they are psychically communicating with your higher self who is informing them of the relevant memories contained within your DNA; they are not reading your history from the Akashic as the Akashic does not record personal memories." What your higher self wants you to know, you will know in the right time and not before. After all, why come all this way to know the ending of your story before it is finished?

Today, more and more children are remembering the bigger soul picture without needing an intuitive translator of the records. These children have been featured in documentaries and books.[366] They recall their former names, their former birthplaces, and names of previous family members. They often recall their entire life in detail, which can be verified through documentation and family members who still live. When they share their memories with us, they let us know that everything happens in divine order and that we all belong to one big soul group. We only have to be available to see and listen, learn and grow.

Chapter Sixteen

FINDING CENTER

Humpty Dumpty sat on a wall.
Humpty Dumpty had a great fall.
All the king's horses and all the king's men.
Couldn't put Humpty together again.

~Nursery Rhyme

No one is immune to the Humpty Dumpty Syndrome. In fact this metaphor is used throughout the medical subspecialties of neurology, psychology, orthopedics, and trauma surgery. When the body or mind becomes injured, it forces you to stop what you're doing and listen to its wisdom. The pain offers a gift in disguise because it means that it is time to focus on you.

It is never easy to be told to stop doing something or alternatively to let something go, even if it's your own body telling you. When the walls come down, the ego cracks. While sitting on the wall of indecision and fear had its comfort level, when we experience the great fall into darkness we are suddenly forced to make a decision. The outcome isn't as bad as we feared. The fall serves to split open the shell and release the buried feelings and pressures. The cracks serve to allow the light to seep through. Our defenses and self-limiting beliefs must crumble and the ego must be shattered in order to open to our true nature and the light of our higher selves. No authority figure or horsepower or men's laws can reconstruct the shell of order when we finally discover the source of true individual power and allow our spirituality to shine.

In his book *She: Understanding Feminine Psychology*, author Robert Johnson characterizes the great fall using the mythology of Psyche and Eros:

"Psyche immediately wants to drown herself in a river. As she faces each of a series of difficult tasks, Psyche wants to kill herself. Does this not point toward a kind of self-sacrifice, the relinquishing of one level of consciousness for another? Almost always in the human experience, the urge toward suicide signals an edge of a new level of consciousness. If you can kill the right thing - the old way of adaptation - and not injure yourself, a new energy-filled era will begin ...Paradox heaped upon paradox, she may find that she did embrace death in her marriage; yes, death to an old way of living."

The key to finding your center is let go of the story you have created about a diagnosis, which gives it power. Never own a disease or allow it to take up space in your consciousness. In his book *Peace With Cancer*, shamanic counselor and mediator Myron Eschowsky suggests a simple and powerful way to center yourself through modeling concepts of Akido, the Japanese martial arts form.[367] Place your hands on your solar plexus, about two inches below the belly button, then breathe and focus attention into your hands. Energy follows attention. When connected to your center, Eschowsky says you cannot be easily budged from your spot. Akido teaches when centered, you are connected to Earth and sky. You are grounded. If you can let go and separate yourself from the drama and energy of the diagnosis, you defuse the emotion. You are seeded in your power. Now when you think about the diagnosis from center, you can focus on healing.

As you let go of the ego's mental musings, the energetic strings can be cut to allow any anger, suffering, or anxiety to simply melt away. This can also be practiced in relationships as compassionate detachment. Compassionate detachment allows you to free yourself of the responsibility for others while you support them so they find their own answers on their path. It allows you to step back as an observer and detach from the outcome in order for the situation to resolve naturally. Attachment is not love. It comes from fear and dependency. It seeks what others can give you rather than what you have to offer.

"Detachment is not that you should own nothing. But that nothing should own you."

~Ali ibn abi Talib

Finding and holding your center is found in loving yourself and in loving others without giving your self away in the process. What you can give to others is possible because you are already full. When you find your center, the ego is freed so you stand strong in your own truth.

Ground and Meditate

Grounding means to "hold your ground." Instead of allowing that spacey feeling to take you away, you stay connected and present. Grounding is about being in your body and maintaining a space for stability. Once grounded, you can better quiet the mind. However, quieting the mind is not as easy as it sounds. The nature of the mind is a revolving door of thoughts that come and go on a continuous basis. The goal is, therefore, not to empty the mind but to: 1) slow the revolving door; 2) appreciate the nature of thought; 3) see the patterns we repeat; and 4) gain an awareness of the nature of the mind. Gaining insight into the mind can be challenging. Like mastering an instrument, a language or a sport, it takes practice.

Once you are able to slow down your thought process, simply listen for what comes next. You may not know what to do at first. But knowing the outcome is not the goal. There is nothing "to do." There is no agenda. Simply relax in this new space. Become aware of your breath and let Spirit guide you. Trust that your experience is the right experience. The more you practice in small spurts the more comfortable you become. The more comfortable you become the longer your practice will be. The answers will come when you are ready to receive them.

To ground yourself for meditation, you can sit in a chair or stand on the grass. You can visualize that your feet grow roots straight into the ground. You can direct a beam of light from your first chakra into the core of the Earth. You also open the crown chakra to allow energy to enter from above. Too much Earth energy can create heaviness or depression when not balanced properly. Like being centered, true grounding means you are open to both Earth and sky energies. Create the visual image that resonates with your inner artist. See the energy travel up and down through your body to fill your heart, then expand the light energy of your biofield outward to the Earth and as far as you like.

You can also choose stones from Nature (with the owner's permission) or choose a special crystal, using your intention to move its energetic vibration down the body and through the feet to connect with the Earth. Using the sacred geometry of a crystal grid is a way to configure and align crystals with your intention to create a pattern of highly focused and ordered energy, a vortex of life force energy that reflects the molecular structure and order of the crystals themselves. In her e-book *The Amazing Power of Crystals*, Reiki Master Elmarie Swartz writes, "The crystals can create a gateway through which energy flows, and that energy is the force which gives birth to all things."[368]

Once grounded you can begin meditation. Meditation is a state of surrender to silence. It is the act of letting go and of finding stillness. Meditation places your focus on the breath, or *prana*; the life force that moves through you to create an internal space apart from your external environment. Your connection to your breath is integral to all types of meditation since the breath is connected to emotions. Shallow breathing happens in the lungs and chest during times of anxiety, anger, and excitement. Long deep breathing draws air deep into the lungs and abdomen, which happens when you are relaxed, peaceful, and happy. By slowing and deepening the breath, you push stale air out from the base of the lungs and bring more oxygen to the blood, which feed your cells. You release stress and relax your body.

"If you want to know something go elsewhere.
If you want to un-know everything then sit and listen."

~Adyashanti, author, spiritual teacher

When we meditate and pray we naturally raise our awareness and our consciousness. As greater numbers of people come together with higher awareness, profound changes on the Earth occur. Such change has been scientifically documented by the HeartMath Institute and others showing that when a large group of people meditate with heart-focused intention, physical reality is altered. A demonstration project led by John Hagelin, professor of Maharishi University in 1993, predicted that a large number of practicing meditators would lower the severe summer crime rate in Washington D.C.[369]

Between June and July of 1993, a group attaining a total of 4,000 meditators came together. When the group reached 2,500, halfway through the period, a statistically significant drop in violence (twenty-five percent) was observed (controlling for weather and other factors). A similar experiment was conducted during the peak of the Israel-Lebanon war in the 1980s that showed an eighty percent drop in the level of violence when the numbers of meditators were largest (600-800 meditators).[370]

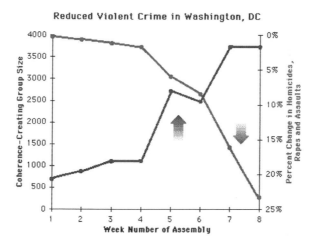

Hagelin says similar studies show similar results, including side effects for people within the geographic vicinity of the mediators – "increased EEG coherence, reduced plasma cortisol, increased blood serotonin levels, biochemical changes, and neurophysiological changes – as if they were meditating."[371]

Results of studies showing the effects of third-party prayer for hospitalized patients have been mixed, with some showing expected beneficial results while others showing the opposite. Many question whether the effects of prayer can be adequately measured using conventional scientific methods since the control groups (who were not actively prayed for) believed their loved ones were praying for them and the majority of participants believed in the effects of spiritual healing.[372]

The Maharishi Effect, predicted by Maharishi Mahesh Yogi over thirty years ago, postulates that world peace is achievable when the square root of one percent of the population –as few as 7,000 people – is heart-focused with the same intention while practicing Transcendental Meditation. Based in the laws of Nature and coherence as described by quantum field theory, our collective consciousness is the unified field that creates this possibility. The unified field influences events distantly and simultaneously, faster than the speed of light. Quantum science suggests that if what we want is world peace, we can have it as soon as we decide. "If something as primitive as a TV set can detect influence from thousands of miles away, why not the human nervous system with its own power grid network?"[373]

Thirty years and five hundred meditation studies later[374] crime has not yet ceased and wars continue. Perhaps heart-focused intention must become a way of life instead of a three-month demonstration project for peace to take hold. However, what the experiment did show is that meditation makes us aware that we are surrounded by an infinite and unconditional love. Mediation opens doors that take us to that home where we can connect to our ageless, higher selves. Meditation is an opportunity to open to our awareness and *listen* to the Source of who we are so we can hear our truth. We receive powerful insights that help us channel our energy in a positive direction. Our short-term and long-term goals are illuminated. We realize that there are no blocks and no limits to what we can accomplish. We see we are full of light and eternal. Simply by reconnecting to Source, we reconnect to ourselves and to each other. To reveal the answers that no one else can give, we need simply go within.

> *"Meditation is not a method but the state of consciousness that you achieve, a place without duality or polarity, a state of presence."*
>
> *~Eckhart Tolle*

There is no cookie-cutter answer that defines meditation. Walking, running, being in Nature, camping, hiking, yoga, Tai Chi, creating poetry or music dancing, listening to music are all forms of meditation. By practicing pranayama, you travel deeper within yourself. With each deep breath, you regenerate yourself and literally slow the aging process. You dial up the flow of energy through the chakras. Ultimately, you gain a greater degree of control over your life.

Meditation moves you into the present moment. Positioning your hands in prayer moudra – thumbs touching fingertip – is another way to enhance awareness. *Mudra* means position or attitude and is more than symbolic. Mudras create specific circuits in the nervous system to increase blood flow to the brain and activate energy flows. Likewise, pressing your thumbs to the center of the chest brings awareness into the heart center.

Meditation and prayer balances your parasympathetic (craniosacral) nervous system, which is active while sleeping, with the sympathetic nervous system, which is active while awake. These tools focus the mind by filtering out concerns and worries of the parasympathetic system that attempt to convince you that its too boring to be silent. When the mind is cleared of chatter, the self-healing process is amplified. When you are focused, you receive insights about your life. One of the miracles of meditation is that we are able to conquer fears, break old patterns, and heal internal suffering. During meditation, the heart, brain, mind, and emotions are balanced and operating in sync, or heart coherence.

Be Present

To be centered in the moment is to be present. During meditation, if you find that your thoughts slip into the past or future, don't judge yourself. Instead, become aware of it and move back into your breath. Be kind to yourself. Focusing the mind in this way takes practice.

> *"Layer by layer I removed all that I thought I was, all that I thought I had to be and in the moment I was left standing naked and vulnerable without identities and labels, I remembered, I am that I am."*
>
> *~Lenita Vangellis, author "Ashanti's Symphony"*

When the mind goes quiet and a sense of peace envelopes you then you have found your center. Space expands and time stands still. David R. Hawkins in his book, *Truth vs. Falsehood* writes, "Because the experience of time stops, there is no apprehension or regret, no pain, no anticipation; the source of joy is unending and ever present. With no beginning or ending, there is no loss or grief or desire. Nothing needs to be done; everything is already perfect and complete. When time stops, all problems disappear; they are merely artifacts of a point of perception. As the Presence prevails, there is no further identification with the body or mind. When the mind grows silent, the thought I AM also disappears and Pure Awareness shines forth to illuminate what one is, was, and always will be, beyond all worlds and all universes, beyond time, and therefore, without beginning or end."

People who achieve such a state of awareness do so by being compassionate towards everything including themselves and their own thoughts. They surrender desire and personal will for that of the greatest good. Many will not attempt to achieve this state of awareness because the steps are too simple. The key is simplicity without distraction and being comfortable in the silence.

Being aware and present takes advantage of the Law of Attraction to work in your favor. Instead of forcing or pushing, you simply allow. You can draw new people and situations into your life by altering the foundation of your beliefs. Change a fearful belief to one of trust. The way to become one with the universe is to trust it to work on your behalf. As you change your thoughts and beliefs, you give the world a new broadcast. If you don't like what you're receiving, simply change your signal. No one else has the power to make you happy. You simply create it for yourself in your own mind, with your own thoughts, and in your own actions.

Practice Makes Presence

Like anything else, living in the moment takes practice and patience. You focus on being exactly where you are in this moment… and now in this moment. Paramahansa Yogananda, an Indian Yogi master who brought Eastern spiritual wisdom, science, and teachings to the West said, "Live each moment completely and the future will take care of itself. Fully enjoy the wonder and beauty of each moment."

"To dwell in the here and now does not mean you never think about the past or responsibly plan for the future. The idea is simply not to allow yourself to get lost in regrets about the past or worries about the future. If you are firmly grounded in the present moment, the past can be an object of inquiry, the object of your mindfulness and concentration. You can attain many insights by looking into the past. But you are still grounded in the present moment."

~Thich Nhat Hanh, Zen Master

Living in the now is a conscious act that requires be-ing within your environment. Instead of strolling aimlessly, you breathe in the beauty of your surroundings, smell the air, listen to the sounds, see the light reflecting off the trees and buildings, look at the pattern of the birds in the yard and how they interact with the squirrel in the tree that has also noticed you. Tilt your head to see a new perspective of the area. Realize that you have also been observed. You will see things you could not see before.

Being present means you are firmly grounded, whether you are writing, dancing, filming, teaching, acting, singing, speaking, listening to music, playing an instrument, gardening, cooking, painting, knitting, etc. When you create in the moment, you do not notice time. You are enraptured by the movement and flow of your creation and transported to a place with no boundaries. You are filled up.

While you may lose your sense of time living in the moment, you also *make* time. You are present to what is around you. When you walk your dog, you stop to talk with your neighbor. When you listen to a friend, you hear what she says. You are not texting someone else on your cell phone. You connect to the ones in front of you. You look them in the eyes. You respect and acknowledge them. In turn, they will be more likely to embrace what you have to say.

Time is a Wave

Grounding allows you to travel to the lower, root vibrations. In an October 1, 2013 radio interview Energy Master Michael Monk refers to the deeper vibrations as the energy of time. Time in this reality is really just a master wave or, in the language of harmonics, a primary tone that creates harmonic overtones of a lighter frequency and a lesser amplitude. In the same way a low A-note on a piano creates a higher A-overtone, the lighter dimensions beyond the third dimension represent overtones to the primary tone on Earth. Time is a vibration, a standing wave that goes in and out at the same time.[375]

"The only reason for time is so that everything doesn't happen at once."

~Albert Einstein

Monks says that few people explore this deeper vibration since all the hype in the spiritual community is about raising vibration and going up, up, up. In the third dimension, depending on the perspective of the collective consciousness, the wave will either face us or not. Currently, consciousness perceives that we face toward the inward pulse of time – toward receiving it. From this viewpoint, we perceive that every event we experience is the universe happening to us, bombarding us with endless hard lessons to teach us. But we are simply standing on one side of time. By coming closer to the zero point, Monk's experience is that you accelerate your consciousness and time begins to come out of you. You begin to manifest in the physical any thought that you hold in your ego.

Finding your center is your ability to connect to the energy that spins through you and connects you to Source. All matter and motion comes down to atomic spin. Each atom spins at a specific rate or vibration, which defines its true nature. Spin is defined by science as torque – the twisting force of an object about an axis. To the human sense of sight, spin is a spiral to which all of Nature conforms, from tornadoes to conch shells to our own galaxy. At the equator, the Earth spins 10,038 miles per hour while moving through space at 67,000 miles per hour. Everything in the universe is spinning. Spin generates symmetry and equilibrium.

"We are not going in circles, we are going upwards. The path is a spiral; we have already climbed many steps."

~Hermann Hesse, poet, novelist, painter

Where you find equilibrium, you find center. Where you find center, you find peace. Where you find peace, you find purpose. In the eye of the storm, confusion changes to clarity. In rediscovering the true center of your being, you find balance. You blossom. You re-Nature.

Though world suffering has always existed in this reality, many are especially sensitive to it now. Taking on the weight of world can make you feel vulnerable and hopeless. While you cannot control the events spinning around you, you can control your own mind. Things only seem hopeless until you reset the mind to the positive and tune out the negative. You always have a choice. You can either spin with the chaos or separate yourself from it. You can either resist or allow.

Peace for our world begins with us, both in how we perceive and react to world events. We have the means at our disposal. Once we declare what we do not want, we become clear about what we do want. Once we can let go of the things we cannot control, we see what we can control. We cannot control the world production of fossil fuels but we can control the demand for it by choosing other sources like biofuels such as solar energy, or hemp, a plant first grown in China around 6,000 BC. We may not have a say in the federal approval of GMO foods but we do have a choice in where we spend our money and in how we grow our own food.

"If you want peace of mind, stop fighting with your thoughts.

~Peter McWilliams, author "Life"

Turn off the TV and channel love. Pollinate optimism by offering a kind word. Nurture the matrix of the Earth by forming rooftop gardens, backyard, vacant lot gardens, and community gardens. Changing the world starts with you in your own neighborhood. When you shift your frequency from fear to love, when you nourish relationships and build health from the ground up, you practice your spirituality.

It is important not to judge yourself when feeling disoriented or disconnected, whether in your own world or the world at large. Simply ground yourself through the first chakra, go within to your silent sanctuary through meditation or prayer, find your zero point, and shift your focus from lack to love. Surrender the hard shell of the ego to the soft wisdom of your spirit.

Chapter Seventeen

SHIFT HAPPENS

When we follow the nudge of spirit's guidance, we cannot help but raise our level of awareness on the path to oneness. This is the path of soul growth. At each new level, one experiences a shift of consciousness, a new way of seeing and a new way of being. A Map of Consciousness was created by Dr. David Hawkins, M.D., a psychiatrist who, himself, experienced several life-altering events. With each event, he noticed a change in his state of consciousness from an ego-based mindset to a state of overwhelming bliss he described as a constant, steady connection with Source.

Levels of Consciousness
Source: Dr. David Hawkins

The Map of Consciousness

The Map of Consciousness illustrates that different levels of consciousness have different levels of power. This numerical log scale spans from 0 to 1,000 where 1 represents the level of a cell and 1,000 + represents the level of an Avatar, Christ, Krishna, and the angelic realms.[376]

Dr. Hawkins' map reflects that every word, every thought, and every intention creates a vibration through the attractor field and that this energy field can be measured by the established science of kinesiology. Kinesiology is the study of muscles and their movements, and first gained attention in the 1960s from the pioneering work of Dr. George Goodheart who discovered, through applied kinesiology, that stimuli such as vitamin and mineral supplements increased the strength of certain indicator muscles, while hostile stimuli such as toxins caused those muscles to suddenly weaken.

In the late 1970s, Dr. John Diamond, in his book *The Body Doesn't Lie*, refined this specialty into Behavioral Kinesiology where indicator muscles would strengthen or weaken in the presence of positive or negative physical, emotional and intellectual stimuli.

Dr. Hawkins' research took Dr. Diamond's technique further in his discovery that this kinesiologic measurement tool could also separate truth from falsehood. Hawkins' Map of Consciousness is described as a scale of the ego with the fulcrum set at the level of 200 representing truth. At a level greater than 200 (true), the arm is strong while below 200 (untrue), the arm is weak. This level is said to indicate the point at which one breaks free of the ego to seek truths for inner growth. Interestingly, testers and test subjects must each calibrate over 200 for accurate results.

The scale is based on twenty years of research and millions of calibrations of truth from statements, thoughts, photos, art, music, politics, religion, and world leaders in every discipline to reflect the human condition.

The kinesiological test, also called reflex nutritional assessment (RNA), used today by Naturopaths, Chiropractors, and other holistic practitioners is one tool that can determine an individual's health status. Using meridian points of traditional Chinese medicine, the tester can assess the percent functionality of organs, one's level of energy, and whether the body is fighting a viral or bacterial infection, to determine in what part of the body there is imbalance. The meridians represent vortices of energy (wheels of light) located midway between the circulatory and nervous systems to affect both the ethereal parts of the body, such as the psyche, and the physical body.[377] Kinesiology testing taps into the life force energy as it moves from the meridians into both directions to serve the body's needs.

Kinesiology testing allows for a customized match between the vibration of the individual's body and the vibration of a natural remedy in order to come into balance. It makes use of the frequency principles espoused by early naturopaths Victor Rocine and Carey Reams. Essential oils, flower essences, homeopathics, herbs, foods, and even crystals naturally access the meridians to create balance. Other modes of natural healing that access this energetic system include acupuncture, EFT, reiki, meditation, Rife frequencies, and others. All affect life force energy.

Today, there are diagnostic machines that measure the body's energetic signatures in the same way muscle testing does, with greater efficiency. Using handheld electrodes, electrodermal testing picks up frequency imbalances that correspond to physical abnormalities. The energy signature of inflammation is identified long before conventional tests can locate it. Electrodermal testing was first developed in the 1950s by Reinhold Voll, is used extensively in Germany, and is being becoming more popular in the United States, with several machines now FDA-approved.

Kinesiology can also identify the right foods for the body since some rates of vibration are healthy and others are not. Processed sugar and altered foods (Aspartame®, Neotame®, colorings, flavorings, MSG, GMOs) not grown according to Nature's laws will vibrate at low frequencies and lead to low vibrational or diseased states in the body. Health and disease naturally reflect different states of vibration within the body. In the same way, music, color, thoughts, words, and people reflect either harmonious or unharmonious vibrations in our biofield.

Muscle testing like RNA has not been reviewed or approved by the FDA nor any other federal health agency. For that matter, the FDA has not approved the contents of this book. ☺ Kinesiology as a means to assess health status has been criticized by mainstream medicine due to lack of controlled data and the reliability of the practitioner. However, mainstream medicine also does not recognize the naturopathic premise that each person is unique or that mind and body and spirit are united as one. In fact, several studies on the effectiveness of RNA continue to be ignored. [378] [379, 380] How electromagnetic energy works in biological systems is also still not fully understood or appreciated by the medical scientific community even though its members accept that this same energy holds atoms together and travels at least as fast as the speed of light.

The kinesiology test cannot be used to foretell the future insofar as the future is created in each moment, but the body can sometimes provide an estimate for each level of healing out a few weeks. Otherwise there are no limits to what can be known using kinesiology testing since consciousness is an energy field of nonlinear domain, not limited by time and space. This non-dimensional realm contains all truths about anything that has ever existed, therefore the answers are not dependent on the belief systems of either the tester or the test subject and therefore are verifiable and repeatable.

According to Hawkins, consciousness knows only truth because only truth exists in reality. It does not respond to falsehood because falsehood is not the opposite of truth. Falsehood is merely a lack or absence of truth, just as cold is the absence of warmth and disease is the absence of health. Remember, health is the body's natural state. Disease merely reflects the body's natural condition in response to a toxin, a deficiency or both. The kinesiology test will not respond to dishonest or egocentric questions related to horse races or the lottery and it will not respond to questions about others' private situations unless they give permission to know the answer.

The scale works equally well with the different range of emotions we all experience. Dr. Bradley Nelson, author of *The Emotion Code*, teaches that when emotions get trapped in a certain organ, the organ begins to resonate at the frequency of that particular emotion. In Hawkins' consciousness scale, trapped emotions at a frequency below 200 represent guilt/shame hate, Apathy, grief, fear, desire, anger and pride. These are ego states that contribute to an overall weakening of the body. The levels between 200 -500 reflect courage, neutrality, willingness, acceptance, and reason. These levels align more directly with truth. The level 500-599 defines a state of pure unconditional love, the state in which we are in complete harmony with our body and our environment. Everything is seen as one. Hawkins found that only 4 percent of the world's population reaches the level of 500 and only 0.4 percent reach level of 540.

Tools of Freedom

Using consciousness as a scale of measurement shows us there is no longer a need to feel trapped within a system that does not get to the root of a problem. By identifying trapped emotions or nutritional imbalances based on a truth scale of consciousness we have the tools to free ourselves. We no longer need to depend on others' expert opinions because we are the answer. Accepting that health is our natural state overcomes the fear of disease. We can don our superhero cape. We are the Alpha and the Omega. We are the problem and the solution. We are the technology we've been waiting for.

Kinesiology as personal tool to self-assessment of health far outpaces lesser scales of measurement. We now have a tool to assess health that makes the old paradigm, of which Buckminster Fuller spoke, obsolete. The truth can be known immediately if we only know how to access it. The truth is that no one else can fix us but us. All we need to access is our own frequency to identify our resonance level on the scale and allow the body to find balance and truth with itself and its environment through Nature.

Tools to Shift Awareness

The way to a new level of health lies in opening to our own awareness. For thousands of years, ancient cultures used all forms of sound vibration not only to induce a feel-good, deep state of relaxation – through chanting, singing, singing bowls, finger chimes, throat singing, instruments, and drumming – but also to raise consciousness.

Music is medicine for the soul. Harmonies and rhythms in music induce emotional states to stimulate and heal the astral and emotional subtle bodies.[381] Music organizes and changes brainwaves by linking body and brain, as demonstrated by EEG measurements in comatose patients.[382] Music with voice is known to reduce stress, calm thoughts, and support the endocrine system.[383]

Today, science accepts that using a binaural beat – sending two different Hertz (Hz) frequencies to each ear – causes both hemispheres of the brain to work in unison and become synchronized, which allows the brain to function at a higher level and create altered states of consciousness.[384]

Drumming is a meditation-prayer tool that anyone can use to open awareness. It has a long tradition in Native American and indigenous cultures as a powerful spiritual tool. Drum circles are still used by Native Americans in ceremonies for healing, initiation, hunt, harvest, and in pow-wows. The traditional drumbeat is a heartbeat. This beat symbolizes the heartbeat of the tribe or the heartbeat of Mother Earth. When used by native shamans in healing, drumming has been shown to produce the same resonating frequency as the Earth (180 cycles per second as measured scientifically). The healing technique of drumming has been practiced by many cultures for thousands of years, from the Minianka healers of West Africa to the shamans of the Tuva Republic in Mongolia. The art of throat singing also originates from the Tuva culture. Throat singing produces a vibration from sounds made in the top and bottom of the throat using nasal sounds, whistling, chest whistling, and lip movements.

Yoga, chanting, breathing, and mantras have been practiced for thousands of years for self-healing. The ancient Hindu scriptures known as the Vedas declared that whoever knows the syllable "Om" obtains all that he desires, especially the desire for knowledge and wisdom. The sound AUM is the sound of I AM, the sound of the sun – 124 Hz – and the sound of light.[385] It evokes the eternal Self, which is our real being.[386] The sound represents the three psychological states of awakening, dreaming, and sleeping, and the transcendent fourth state of illumination. Another teaching of the Upanishad says that we should meditate on this symbol and by doing so we come to omniscience, united with all.[387]

As the most ancient form of yoga, Kundalini Yoga is considered the king of yogas. The word kundalini means "awareness." Practiced for thousands of years in an unbroken tradition, kundalini yoga combines the physical and spiritual. It provides one way to encounter yourself within a very short time. With thousands of meditations and kriyas, anyone can partake. No matter what condition your body, mind, or emotions are in, Kundalini can be one tool that opens you to the challenge that informs you about your life. Eyes are closed and focused on the third eye (brow line) to stimulate the pituitary gland. The pituitary, (the Seat of Intuition), is the master gland which regulates the body's functions. It communicates with the pineal gland (the Seat of the Soul) which has the Master Plan. The interaction between the two glands brings stillness and clarity, the experience of True Self. Physiologically, it is the brain telling itself how to regulate itself.

In many people this connection is blocked and the glands do not talk to each other. The pineal gland can become calcified from fluoride (found in municipal water and drugs). Without a direct plan from the pineal gland, the pituitary looks for something else to stimulate it and give it direction (alcohol, drugs, caffeine, sugar, sex), and can become the Seat of Addiction. Kundalini yoga helps redirect the connection between these two glands.[388] All Kriyas serve to reset body and mind as well as connect us to the divine as has been practiced for thousands of years. Kundalini teaches a flexible spine is a flexible mind.

As a body-mind-spiritual workout, Kundalini stimulates energetic and immune systems, balances brain hemispheres and resets body rhythms. The Kriya Yoga technique is a pranayama (deep breathing), a scientifically proven tool that nourishes the body and activates the parasympathetic nervous system to decrease blood pressure, respiratory rate, heart rate, and baseline oxygen consumption.[389]

"Offering the inhaling breath into the exhaling breath and offering the exhaling breath into the inhaling breath, the yogi neutralizes both breaths; thus he realizes prana from the heart and brings life force under his control."

~The Bhagavad Gita IV:29

The Breath (Pranayama)

In esoteric terms, pranayama transmutes the breath into subtle life force energy and awakens awareness to your higher self.[390] India yogi Sri Yukteswar taught "The ancient yogis discovered that the secret of cosmic consciousness is intimately linked with mastering the breath." In practice of this technique, a practitioner not only breathes, but holds his attention on the act of breathing which focuses concentration. Focus on breath takes attention away from worries and serves to de-stress and relax the body.[391] The body is oxygenated at the cellular level, reinforcing subtle energy currents in the spine, which affect the cerebrospinal centers along the entire chakra system.

Long deep breathing, breath of fire, and nostril breathing are among the most common paranyama techniques to synchronize right and left brain hemispheres. Long, slow, deep breathing is activated using the belly as a bellows as you focus to fill the lower abdominal area first and then fill the diaphragm Exhale by moving the belly in first to push air out of the bottom of the lungs. Filling the lungs to capacity feeds your electromagnetic field and pumps spinal fluid to the brain, bringing greater energy. It regulates the body's pH, stimulates production of endorphins in the brain, cleanses nerve channels, helps release blocks in meridian energy flow, and restores the aura.

Breath of fire is a light, fast, rhythmic breath through the nose, mouth closed, with the abdomen acting like a bellows to pump the breath. Breath of Fire oxygenates the blood at a high rate. It boosts the nervous system, causing the glands to secrete and purify the blood. Two minutes of yoga using breath of fire is equal to two hours of regular exercise for oxygenation and metabolic benefits.

In nostril breathing, the left nostril is tied to relaxation. It reflects the moon's energy – reflective, calming, cooling, female. Inhaling through the left nostril stimulates the brain's capacity to reset your framework of thinking and feeling, allowing new perspectives.[392] The right nostril has energizing properties. It reflects the energy of the sun – bright, fiery, awakening, male. Exhaling through the right nostril relaxes the thinking brain and helps to break automatic patterns. As we tend to breathe predominantly out of one nostril, alternate nostril breathing brings equal amounts of oxygen to both sides of the brain for improved clarity and brain function. You remove stale air while cooling, calming, and nourishing the brain. After only two minutes of focused breathing, you can feel a distinct difference in wellbeing. Practice this to relax before a stressful event or before bed to promote calm.

Nostril Breathing Technique:

- Sit with spine straight and shoulders down with eyes closed and focused at brow point.
- Close the right nostril with your right thumb. Let the rest of your fingers point toward the sky.
- Inhale through the left nostril then turn your hand and close the left nostril with the right pinky and exhale through the right side.
- Inhale through the right nostril (always inhale through the nostril that you have just exhaled with). Close with the right thumb and exhale through the left nostril. Inhale through the left nostril and continue for 2 to 10 minutes.

The Kriya Yogi who practices kundalini yoga mentally directs kundalini – life force energy – which is coiled like a serpent at the base of the spine. In this ancient Hindu practice, life energy spirals upward and downward around the six spinal centers (medullary, cervical, dorsal, lumbar, sacral, and coccygeal plexuses). The six spinal centers (twelve by polarity) are considered inner constellations which are said to revolve around the sun of the third eye. In this way, the inner universe reflects the outer universe of the twelve astral signs of the zodiac, the Cosmic Man.

In Kriya yoga, sexual energy of the root chakra is transmuted into spiritual energy of the higher crown chakra. The serpentine energy corresponds to an energetic unwinding of the DNA helix and the release of DNA codes in a transfer of Earth wisdom back to the people. As energy moves from the lower chakras to the third eye (forehead) one is able to create what one visualizes. In this way, sexual energy is channeled and used to heal the body, improve relationships, enhance productivity, and create success.

Yoga helps one to see things in relation to one's greatest potential, to see oneself and all things as aspects of a greater reality. According to Paramahansa Yogandanda, Kriya yoga is the same science known by Krishna, Patanjali (one author of the yoga sutras), Christ, St. John, St. Paul, and other disciples. Jesus not only knew yoga but, like the masters of the East, he taught yoga to his closest disciples. The original teachings of Jesus showed that he taught a unifying path which brings all seekers to the kingdom of God.[393] Yogis believe that that one half-minute of Kriya equals one year of natural spiritual unfoldment. After years of successful practice, the body of the advanced Kriya Yogi can achieve such lightness that the body actually levitates.[394]

Mantras are more than Sanskrit healing words. Like the sound Om, mantras are sounds of a predetermined vibratory effect with known powerful physiologic and mental effects on the body and the chakras. This is because the hard palate in your mouth contains fifty-eight energy points that connect to all your body's physical systems. It is not necessary to know the meaning of the words to affect healing. The sounds themselves, whether whispered or repeated aloud, stimulate these points to activate and repattern the energy of your entire chakra system. The most basic mantra of Kundalini yoga is Sat Nam, or True Self. The True Self is the highest frequency, your essence, the infinite you that never changes.

"Mantras are not small things, mantras have power. They are the mind vibration in relationship to the Cosmos. The science of mantra is based on the knowledge that sound is a form of energy having structure, power, and a definite predictable effect on the chakras and the human psyche."

~Yogi Bhajan

Rebalance Thyroid and Heart: The Sa Ta Na Ma chant is a Kirtan Kriya that rebalances the entire endocrine system. The words sa (life) ta (death) na (rebirth) ma (existence) are the primordial sounds common to every language in the world.[395] Using mudras (hand gestures) in combination with mantra serves balance the thyroid if this twenty-minute exercise is done consecutively for forty days. Any break in the cycle means you must start again from the beginning, but once finished, the effects are known to last indefinitely.[396]

Likewise, the Jot Kriya can help or prevent heart problems. Sit with a straight spine. Press palms of the hands together three inches in front of your face with fingertips at brow level. Let the breath regulate itself. Hold this pose for 1-2 minutes to start and work up to eleven minutes. As with any new exercise, check with your healthcare provider before beginning. Side effects include increased flexibility.

These ancient cultures knew that their spiritual and therapeutic practices created vibrations that brought on feelings of peace. They knew this even without the science that now shows yoga and drumming to rebalance the brain hemispheres by changing brain frequencies from beta waves (focused concentration and activity) to alpha waves (calm and relaxed), and theta waves (psychic states), which are found in deep states of meditation.[397]

The rhythmic vibration of chanting and drumming is being rediscovered around the world for overall wellbeing. Drumming is also used in the practice of Shamanic Journeying, which allows one to journey to altered states while lying comfortably in your home, similar to active/lucid dreaming.[398] The vibration of the drum permeates the entire brain to improve focus and produce endorphins, the body's natural painkillers, to create deep relaxation. Not only does drumming heal neural pathways that may be blocked, but it also boosts the immune system.[399]

The most important thing is to find the style of relaxation that works for you. Whether you walk in Nature, practice yoga, read poetry, chant a mantra, meditate with sound frequencies, dance, or beat a drum, it is your ability to relax that gives you access to the unconscious, intuitive mind. Feelings of insight, love, truth, and understanding beyond ordinary understanding are revealed. And the inner guidance of Source flows easily.

Chapter Eighteen

FINDING HAPPINESS

Comedian, actor, musician Tim Minchin, in his humorous address to the University of West Australia graduating class, bestowed a list of life lessons. Lesson number two: "Don't seek happiness. Happiness is like an orgasm. If you think about it too much it goes away. Keep busy and make someone else happy and you might get some as a side-effect."[400]

While there is much truth in the advice not to "seek" happiness, life should not only be about making others happy. If your happiness depends on what someone else does or how someone else feels, then you are living someone else's life. Life is about sharing *your* happiness. For that to happen, happiness has to start with you.

Copyright 2007 by Randy Glasbergen.
www.glasbergen.com

GLASBERGEN

"Money can't buy happiness, but if I had a big house, fancy car and a giant plasma TV, I wouldn't mind being unhappy!"

Indian guru, Ramana Maharshi observed that people often equate happiness with pleasure gained from external causes and possessions, not realizing that "real happiness is permanent while pleasure is not."[401] Pleasure that ends in pain is misery. However, devoid of possessions there is still the desire for happiness. This desire that arises from within is proof that happiness is a natural, ever-present state of Self.

When it comes to eating for health, the nutrient value of food depends on how well food is absorbed. Absorption is partially determined by psychological factors, like how we feel when we eat food and live life. An anxious eater eats fast. This reduces the release of hormones in the gut that creates the feeling of being full and results in overeating. Anxious eaters also create the "fight or flight" response that puts them in survival mode. To fight or flee, the body releases two hormones: adrenaline to provide energy, and cortisol to increase appetite to replenish lost energy. When we experience chronic stress, we "pack it on" because the body naturally craves simple carbohydrates and sugars.[402] Fear about gaining weight further increases cortisol in the blood, which desensitizes us to pleasure. Fear creates the self-fulfilling prophecy: "If I eat those treats, I won't be able to stop."

Alternatively, being in a state of happiness slows us down, relaxes us and we breathe ourselves into the present moment. When we are happy, endorphins are produced in the brain and digestive system. The connection shows us that our very biochemistry takes healthy pleasure in eating. The body knows inherently what to do for balance and balance is not found in counting calories but in counting your blessings. Marc David, founder of Psychology of Eating writes, "When you're turned on by food, you turn on metabolism. Our nature demonstrates to us how happiness, metabolism, and a naturally controlled appetite are interwoven to the core."[403]

Go Within

Thousands of years ago, Buddha taught that for any given situation in life, if we do not attach ourselves to any outcome but simply go within and align ourselves with divine purpose, then nothing can influence our moods. After all, between the distractions of life and the limits we impose upon ourselves, it may not be possible to conceive of the best possible outcome.

> *"When you discover that all happiness is inside of you, the wanting and needing are over and life gets very exciting."*
>
> *~Byron Katie, author*

Going within, you find that happiness is truly a state of being. On the other hand, no one said that finding bliss would be easy. It may be the hardest work you do because you may have to temporarily lose yourself. You may need to stop lying to yourself and dare to see yourself as worthy. In order to open the gates of the heart and let go of any inferiority complexes you must learn to love and honor yourself. Today, the leader of the Tibetan people, his Holiness the Dalai Lama says, "If you want others to be happy, practice compassion. If you want to be happy, practice compassion."

Before we are born, we know a great, infinite love. As we grow up, we forget. We forget our limitless potential for compassion, love, peace, and happiness. Through reconnecting with the Earth, we have the opportunity to rediscover all of this if we are able to observe that our environment is really a roadmap for what is going on inside of us. It may take some of us longer than others to open the map but if we can reset the GPS, we can take ourselves in a new direction. As the navigator of our journey, *we* decide when we take the next step. It is best to continue the journey not by regretting where we've been or worrying about where we're headed, but by just being cool about where we are right now. That is likely what the ancient Tibetans would tell us if they were here now.

Dreams, Signs, and Synchronicities

When you are aware of the moment, you are in the flow. Being in the flow of life is where the current is smoothest. If you are unsure about where you are as you go about your day, ask for a specific sign for guidance. For some, seeing a hawk reassures them they are on the right path. If you choose to request a sign, choose something that you are likely to see on any given day, like a coin turned on its head, or a special flower. If you request a rose, be open to the sign showing up as the real thing or perhaps on a billboard or in the lyrics of a song. Anything is possible.

Alternatively, not seeing what you want to see may also be a sign. Constantly coming up against challenges or blocks in life is a sign to stop what you are doing, turn around, and go a different way. Once you choose to be present in the moment, you create a space for new experiences to happen. You open new doors. You allow for new people to come into your life. Of course, distractions will sometimes take you out of the moment. Don't judge yourself. Just refocus your attention and come back to the moment. When you reconnect to your true self, you can never return to the old ways. Your life becomes a journey forward, to the presence of who you truly are.

American writer Joseph Campbell in his book *The Power of Myth* said, "Follow your bliss" and doors will open to you. The signs are always there, guiding you. Follow your gut instincts, your intuition, your heart, and Source provides signposts along your path. These signs for self-healing can come through dreams, inspiration, synchronicities, imagination, and people. As beings of light vibration, information flows to you in as many different ways – light, sound, feeling – as you are able to receive it.

In his book *The Secret History of Dreaming*, Author Robert Moss writes, "The new approach to health care will feature the healing power of story. In the clear understanding that finding meaning in any life passage may be at the heart of healing, our healers will help people use the power of dreaming to move beyond personal history into a bigger story that contains the juice and sense of purpose to get them through."

Our experience in our linear 3D-reality is an illusion of the limited mind. In dimensions beyond the third, past, present, and future are not sequential but happening simultaneously; in "no-time." In dreams, we are able to access nonlinear time because the mind can perceive events happening at any time in any dimension. We are able to access our simultaneous selves. You only need to be open and aware to receive the messages and gain insight. Signs and symbols come in all forms, as we are able to receive them, and they come from the soul. Theses signs are your inner compass showing you a reference point for where you are in the unfolding of your life story.

Dreams speak the language of symbols connecting you to your higher self. A recurring dream of warning can be precognitive, an opportunity to make changes now to prevent a negative outcome. Dreams can be as clear as traveling on the wrong side of the road or driving a bus you don't know how to operate. Dreams can also provide the truth of a situation in the face of an inaccurate diagnosis. If inconsistencies exist between the opinions of authorities and what your dreams reveal, this presents an opportunity to question and investigate further. Keep a dream journal by writing them down upon awakening for best recall, and watch themes unfold over time.

Other signs come as synchronicities. Perhaps you are thinking about someone and suddenly they call you or you happen to run into them. Or you may be looking for a particular car to purchase and you begin to notice the same car everywhere you go. Maybe every time you look at the clock you see the number eleven. A synchronicity is not a coincidence because you are in control. These symbols merely serve to remind you of your place in the larger plan.

You may perceive the signs around you as positive or negative. Either way, they are meant to direct you as clearly as traffic lights. While some signs may show you are on the right track in your choices, there are also crossroads in life when a bell may sound and a gate comes down to stop you in your tracks. You may fail to find a job. Your health may take a downward spiral. Relationships may drain you or suddenly end, leaving you at a loss. But you are not lost. In his book *The Second Sin*, Psychiatric critic Thomas Szasz M.D. writes, "People often say this or that person has not yet found himself. But the self is not something one finds, it is something one creates."

"Every act of consciousness learning requires the willingness to suffer an injury to one's self esteem. That is why young children, before they are aware of their own self-importance, learn so easily."

~Thomas Szasz, psychiatrist

People come into our lives for "a reason, a season, or a lifetime" to help us create. When the collaboration is done, they may leave or you may leave. It is important to mourn the loss and release it. As you purposefully let go, you make room for new people and experiences to make their way to you.

While no one seeks out negative or unwanted signs, these signs serve to direct you on your path. The universe gives warnings as cosmic wake-up calls even if you may not want to receive them.[404] Yet all things that come your way are part of a perfect plan for your growth, to prompt you to take that next step on your journey. Think of them as yellow or red flashing lights tell you to stop and think before proceeding further.

In terms of health, the reason to "catch a disease" is to figure out how to release it. The catch-and-release fishing metaphor is applicable even in the earliest stages to prevent disease. For instance, you may appreciate food and know where all the best restaurants are. You know not to overindulge but each time you eat a rich meal you experience heartburn (reflux). Instead of listening to your body and altering your diet, you choose to ignore the signs and take a pill for temporary relief based on the opinion of a so-called expert. Before long, you have created a chronic health condition because the pill fails to address the underlying cause of low amounts of stomach acid.

If the reflux goes away upon taking the pill, you likely have too little stomach acid, not too much, causing undigested food to back up into the esophagus. An ideal stomach pH is 2-4. The pill only serves to further drive stomach pH in the wrong direction, toward a more alkaline pH creating poorer digestion and conditions that invite pathogenic microbes (H. pylori) into an area of the body they do not belong and for which you will likely be prescribed a long-term antibiotic.

Instead, you can choose to empower yourself and prevent the problem in the first place. A common folk remedy is to drink one tablespoon apple cider vinegar in a glass of apple juice or water before a meal, or altering the diet altogether. Using a simple home test, people can assess their own stomach acid pH and, if necessary, supplement temporarily with betaine HCL as a replacement for low acid conditions. Betaine HCL is thought to retrain your stomach to get to the correct pH levels over time. Taking just thirty ml a day of honey can also help heal those suffering from gastritis, duodenal ulcers, and stomach ulcers since honey naturally balances stomach acid.[405]

There is always a choice. The signs and solutions have always been at our disposal. We can look to our bodies the body's intelligence for answers just as native cultures looked to animals, cloud formations, and dreams for answers. The Iroquai Seneca Indians still look to dreams for guidance. They've said, "The dream world is the real world."[406] The Egyptians observed how the stars moved across the sky to foretell the future. The Romans interpreted dreams, synchronicities, observed lightning in the sky, and the flight patterns of birds.

Today, as in the past, shamans teach that everything that exists is alive and has a spirit. Shamans know we are equal to everything around us. In every continent, shaman healers still read signs, examine beliefs and fears, and interpret dreams and images to offer their insight. They listen to their surroundings. They perform ceremonies to heal emotional and physical illnesses in respect of the higher elements of Nature. They embody service to others to bring meaning and purpose back to life and to restore balance and harmony back to community.[407] What did all of these cultures over the world and across time have in common? They understood Earth to be a living organism. They saw their world as a web of life where all things are interconnected to Source.

We are each a shaman on a healing journey to find balance and to reconnect to our higher selves to more easily follow spirit. Spirit shows us the reality we create is non-linear and comes through symbols and images. It is another way to receive information about the cause of our dis-ease. Disease forces us to learn. When we are pushed to our limit, we blossom. Observing the signs on our path allows us to make necessary changes to become whole. The answers come are from the heart and are accessible at any moment.

When we reconnect to Nature and her cycles and seasons, we learn that nothing is born and nothing dies. Just because we do not see something or hear something does not mean it does not exist. The TV signal continues to broadcast even if the TV cannot receive the signal.

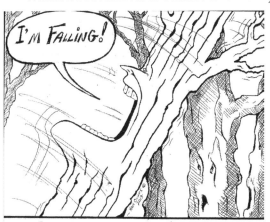

BOB STARTED TO FALL IN THE WOODS...
AND WANTED TO MAKE SURE EVERYONE HEARD!

When we attach to an idea of existence, it makes us think that something exists or does not exist. The Buddha said that when conditions are sufficient something manifests. When conditions fail, it does not. The germ exists only when the environment of the organism is favorable to its growth. An epidemic exists when whole communities come out of balance. Stem cells differentiate into fat cells or muscle cells or bone depending on the influence of their environment. When we perceive our true nature, that we are birthless and deathless, we transcend the fear of death and truly live life. Like Earth's cycles, we cycle through the budding of our Spring, the bloom of our Summer, the looking inward of our Fall, and the destiny of our Winter, where our gifts are given to the community. We are ever evolving, shapeshifting beings.

As long as we have the physical body, the house of our soul on this Earth plane, we should honor, respect, and love it completely. The body is not merely a shell. It speaks to us each moment in subtle and not so subtle ways. We can neglect its wisdom and complain about it in the third person, "I have a bad gallbladder," or we can align with it and come into our own. How well we listen and respond to the body is always a choice, the consequences of which will direct us to the next stop on the journey.

> *"Thanks to our fear of death in this country I won't have to die. I'll pass away."*
>
> *~George Carlin, comedian*

Like all things in life, happiness manifests as soon as you decide. Happiness is not found in measuring possessions on a scale. It is not alien. Happiness is limitless and natural and found within you. When you realize its permanence you consciously reactivate your connection to the Source within you. Happiness reveals itSelf. You rediscover your true nature.

Chapter Nineteen

THE EGO AND THE SPIRIT

Ego says "Once everything falls into place, I will find peace.
Spirit says, "Find peace and everything will fall into place."

~Author Unknown

Where does the ego fit in to spiritual evolution? We have come to hold the ego as the part of us with the least value, defined as the "false center." We label ego as the defensive part of the psyche that fuels all the negatives in the mind, the root cause of all resistance and suffering. We like to blame the ego for everything we don't accept about ourselves. Yet if we came here with everything we needed for this life, then don't we also need the ego?

As individual expressions of the whole, our ego is our point of reference, an awareness of self. It is the thought bubble above your head that thrives on attention and says, "Notice me." It is also a reflection of others.

The reflective nature of ego is expressed in the way that the people who are the most critical of others are often the most self-critical. Those who cannot trust others are themselves untrustworthy. When we judge others, we project what we don't like about ourselves and point out their flaws as we see them. To us, the most irritating people may be complainers or rumor mongers. They may be hypocrites, people who say one thing and do another. They may be know-it-all, conceited, arrogant, pigheaded, egotistical, short-tempered, lazy slobs. And worst of all, long-winded!

But look again. The universe puts those in front of us who echo our thoughts back to us as we send them out. Our fears and jealousies rebound back to us from the souls around us. When we hold tight to these experiences, we embody them. We associate ourselves with the shadow emotions of our past. But we are not our emotions, just as we are not our ego. Fear, like any emotion, is not real. Danger is real. Fear is a product of our thoughts and our perceptions. Fear, like anger or jealousy, is a choice. In the documentary *Shadow Effect*, author Debbie Ford says that if what we hear from others does not affect us, it is likely a projection of the other person and has nothing to do with us. If what we hear does affect us emotionally, it is likely a reflection.[408]

None of us likes to admit we have insecurities. But if we are open, the annoying traits of others show us what we still need to work on in ourselves. They show us our ego. Like attracts like. People who find each other to share love also share mutual problems. Too often, each person in a relationship will blame the other, leave issues unresolved, and move on to the next mate. The pattern is repeated until the owner of the problem admits ownership. In the same way, those who believe they are loved by being needed will attract needy people. Those who believe they are victims will attract an abuser. We continue to draw similar situations again and again, each one more challenging than the last until the lesson is learned, if it ever is.

The problem isn't out there; it is in here. If each admits the problem, each can then focus on giving and receiving love instead of casting blame. One cannot demand love from another without first being willing to give love. Giving love starts with loving yourself. You fill up your own cup first and only then can you give to others. It is no different than aiding others in an airplane emergency scenario. When the oxygen masks come down, you secure your mask first.

The good news is that those qualities we admire most in others – our idols – are also a reflection of us. Our answers are literally staring us in the face. The challenge in spiritual growth is to recognize the ego as a mask we wear to cover up our dark side. We cannot be afraid to embrace and expose the darkness so it can be released. The purpose of the ego is to show us all that we are both light and dark and not to fear the person behind the mask. We must embrace our ordinary self. David R. Hawkins, Ph.D. author of "Power vs. Force" writes, "Just being ordinary in itself is an expression of divinity; the truth of one's real self can be discovered through the pathway of everyday life. To live with care and kindness is all that is necessary. The rest reveals itself in due time. The commonplace and God are not distinct."

We may come into this life with a strong ego where everything comes easily. We may have looks, money, status, fortune, and fame. We may be the go-to person for advice in our profession. But at the same time we may also be secretly nursing an addiction that undercuts our credibility to the core. Alternatively, we may come in with a small ego, feeling worthless where life is a struggle based in self-limiting beliefs. In both cases the challenge is equal – to break through the fear of being ordinary, the fear of not being perfect – to begin the work of becoming our true selves. The level at which we begin with the ego is less important than the healing journey to spirit.

When spirit finally calls, it is time to pay attention. The fall into darkness is the signal. It allows us to gain perspective to see its opposite (lightness) and to not take either for granted. The death of a pet can take us to depths deeper than that of a family member. The emptiness may stop us and shift priorities. Suddenly all the details of life don't seem to matter as much. A light goes on to show us new focus and lead us to ways of being.

Our experiences grow out of contrasting energies, light and dark, fire and ice, ecstasy and depression in order to generate a spark that feeds the creativity of the whole self. Like a hologram, we cannot experience any part of ourselves without experiencing the complete self. We cannot experience pleasure without knowing pain, courage without knowing fear, love without knowing hate, or knowing who we are without knowing who we are not. Our ego and its shadows serve a purpose. Only when we are able to appreciate our shadows do we move out of them.

"What we are here to undertake on earth while immersed in matter is fundamentally a spiritual journey aimed at the growth and perfection of the soul, a journey which may go back to the very origins of what made us human in the first place."

~Graham Hancock, The War on Consciousness, TED Talk

The unification of extreme opposites is seen in all ancient religious texts, from Islamic mysticism (Sufism) to Jewish Kabbalahism to Chinese Taoist tradition to Buddhism to the Gnostic texts to the Bhagavad Gita. All speak of reconciling or transcending pairs of opposites to reach enlightenment. Enlightenment is not a transformation into something more or better. It is the simple awareness of who we already are. Enlightenment is achieved when the lower self is strong and empowered and balanced with the higher self. When we embrace individuality in this way, the ego relaxes to become part of the whole. We are transformed. When we heal ourselves and we are able to help others heal.

In many ways, this is the model of the Twin Flame relationship. Until we have achieved the ability to be one with ourselves, we will never be able to be one with another. Both realities happen without resistance through allowing Nature to take its course. As individual expressions of the whole, the ego is essential in leading us to that point.

The ego and the spirit balance each other. When your passion in life is being drained away, it is your spirit that tells you that something has to change, or the signs will eventually knock you upside the head to capture your attention. Your ego, on the other hand, tells you the opposite – that this is not the time to make any big changes in life. It is the voice that says, "You want to leave your job or your marriage? What else can you do anyway? How are you going to start over at this late stage in the game? Just take the antidepressant and be done with it."

The longest distance is said to be between the head and the heart. But be glad that you can question your ego. The fact that you are having a conversation with the ego-mind tells you that your higher self is in control. The higher self speaks from the heart. But the ego is not the enemy. Ego is part of you. However, it is only one opinion even if it happens to be coming from you. If the mind is clear, you can perceive the differences between them and recognize that you have alternative resources within yourself, outside the ego, which allow you to create a different story.

"The soul always knows what to do to heal itself.
The challenge is to silence the mind."

~Caroline Myss, author and medical intuitive

In all healing journeys practicality does have its place, however there must be room for compassion and love and passion to step in. To attract what you want, tune into the frequency of what you want. Through alignment with self-love you attract situations and people who reflect back your true nature. So be clear about who you are. Make a list, tell yourself out loud, and remember to feel it in your heart. There is no need to look for something or someone. Chasing others is fleeting. In relationships, attracting the right partner is first about being the right partner and letting that person walk into your life. Believe you have everything you need right now and embody that. Feel it at the base of your spine. Then let go of any attachment to the outcome.

By letting go of expectations, you accept without judgment and love without restriction. You become a positive force in the energy dynamic in which you interact. When you can separate yourself from your emotions, you see all relationships as a snap shot for where you are in your unfolding process. The joy you gain from one experience is a gift that propels you forward to new experiences. The movement forward happens for the highest good.

"Expectation is the root of all heartache."

~William Shakespeare, playwright

Boundaries

As a spirit being, it is important to separate your unique energy from the intense emotional energies of others. There are many ways to create energetic boundaries. One way is to simply declare that any energy that is not your own goes back from where it came. Yet even with the best of intentions, people can easily take on other people's emotions without knowing it.

Stressful events and hurtful situations are a part of our lives but we don't have any reason to carry them as toxic emotional baggage. You can be empathetic without becoming emotionally drained. You can serve others without taking on their pain. You can love unconditionally without attachment. Being neutral, free of judgment and compassionate is possible when you take precautions and take responsibility for your energy. However, in large groups you may not know whose energy causes you to feel unbalanced.

If you suffer from headaches when you are at work, you may be feeling others' emotions in your third eye (sixth chakra). When in a large crowd or group you might feel overpowered by a gripping sensation in the center of your abdomen. This is the solar plexus (third chakra), the seat of emotions and your personal power. Being empathic, you are naturally drawn to those who suffer or are bullied, but you don't have to become a dumping ground for their issues and emotions. Incoming emotions from others can lead to digestive disorders and lower back problems. You have the ability to protect yourself by dialing your chakras up or down at will, simply by using your intention and your imagination. It is always important to ground and protect yourself.

Empathic individuals who expose themselves to energy vampires on a regular basis, unknowingly drain themselves. Use your imagination to create some energetic boundaries. Image a protective white light surrounding you that nothing can penetrate. Visualize a virtual set of chainmail, lightweight and strong as steel, to allow the beneficial to flow in while the toxic bounces off. Envision each chakra as an all-seeing glass eye that alerts you well in advance to prevent any negative energies from penetrating. In all relationships, we naturally send out etheric cords to others, but we don't need to maintain these connections long-term.

Energetic cords are neither good nor bad but they do drain our energy over time. At least once a week, consider cleansing your etheric body of any cords you have attached unconsciously to other people, places, or things, as well as cords that may have innocently been attached to you. You can activate a circular breathing pattern by breathing in white light through your root chakra and exhaling it through your crown chakra. You can consciously and without judgment clear cords to take back your power while sending others' energy back. Failure to protect yourself can mean absorbing emotions from others that can eventually lead to addictions (alcohol, drugs, sex, food) or weight gain in order to compensate. Withholding emotions results in building internal barriers that be emotionally crippling, physically destructive, or explosive and projected onto others. You may create an emotional debt so large you lose yourself.

There is no need to declare emotional bankruptcy. Forgive those who have hurt you in the past, bless them, and thank them for the lesson they offered you at that time in your soul's development. Make it your intention to release old hurts to the Earth to be renewed or to the light to be transformed. More importantly, forgive yourself for holding on to the pain for so long. In the space left behind, you as the artist create a blank canvas from which you can paint with new, life-affirming experiences. Don't waste a moment. Empower yourself.

Chapter Twenty

LOVE AND FORGIVENESS

"Love is not a vibration. Love is an interpretation of a vibration. So is fear. A vibration is neutral. It's a wave. It fluctuates. To a fully evolved consciousness you can experience the whole rainbow spectrum and say that they are all love. And if you love them all then you will be radiating all colors from red to violate and they will all be love. The whole idea is to day by day learn to interpret more vibrations as being love. The one and only pathway to experiencing unconditional love is to love all vibrations."

~Michael Monk, energy master

Love is the ultimate power. Love is the heart of the physical universe, the mental universe and the spiritual universe. As your heart beats, so beats your power.

Have a Heart... and another brain

The news just keeps getting better. You are really a being with three brains. The heart, like the gut and the head, possesses its own brain, complete with nervous system, decision-making powers, and a network of neurons and neurotransmitters.[409] The organ that pumps blood to every cell in the body in under a minute also generates the largest electromagnetic field in the body. The electrical field as measured in an electrocardiogram (ECG) is about sixty times greater in amplitude than the brain waves recorded in an electroencephalogram (EEG),[410] yet it emits an energy field five thousands times greater than the brain.

The amazing heart is formed during pregnancy at twenty days and begins to beat at twenty-one to twenty-two days, well before the brain, which begins to develop around six weeks. The ancient Egyptians believed the heart, not the brain, was the source of human wisdom, emotions, memory, the soul, and the personality itself. They felt that the heart linked all the parts of the body together, which is why they ceremoniously embalmed it after death. They threw out the brain. The ancient Greeks and Chinese believed the heart to be the Seat of the Spirit.

The heart is the transmitter that sends the signal of your declaration, if your declaration is pure. In doing so, it acts independently from the cerebral brain in its power to process, think, learn and feel. In its ability to reason, perceive, and emote, the heart has a mind and a language all its own. It communicates with the brain and other organs through its production of hormones and neurotransmitters – dopamine and adrenaline – known to mediate emotions, and therefore also acts as an endocrine gland.[411]

Paul Servan-Schreiber, psychiatrist and author of the book *The Instinct to Heal: Curing Depression, Anxiety and Stress Without Drugs and Without Talk Therapy*, says "There is a constant exchange between the heart and the brain. Research shows that a coherent heart rhythm is able to bring the emotional brain to rest. When your heart is beating in a healthy way, you can heal stress, depression, tension, and other mental afflictions."

Research from the HeartMath Institute shows that the heart transmits love faster than the brain alone transmits thoughts, faster than the speed of light. Heart speed is instantaneous. When you feel love or affection for another, your heartbeat shows up in the other person's magnetic brain rhythm.[412] When you have a high level of heart coherence, the body's cardiovascular, nervous, hormonal, and immune systems run more efficiently and harmoniously. It is the heart, not the brain, that is more important when it comes to illness and health. Emotions are faster and more powerful than thoughts and intentions alone.

Author Gregg Braden, speaking on the power of the heart, says that satellites above the Earth monitoring magnetic fields can pick up spikes of energy precisely at the moment human emotion of the Earth is focused on a natural disaster (e.g., 9-11), documenting that the emotional energy of the heart travels far beyond the body.

Braden says, "These fields are now implicated in everything from the immune response of humans throughout the planet, climate, weather patterns, cycles of war and peace, our ability to solve problems, and our cognitive abilities...all are linked to the magnetic fields of the Earth."[413]

Eckhart Tolle says this healing shift can be brought about through meditation practice with conscious breathing which creates a space to help stop the thinker from being tortured by his own mind. Deepak Chopra describes this head-heart process with the acronym STOP where S = stop thinking, T= take three deep breaths, smiling everywhere in your body, O = observe your body, and P = proceed with love and kindness.[414]

When we understand that we are beings of body, mind, and spirit, we appreciate our creative power to heal ourselves and the planet. Our health is intimately entangled between inner and outer environments. Emotions are processed and absorbed into our consciousness for the soul to digest in the same way that food is processed and absorbed into the bloodstream for the body to digest. What we feed our cells is just as important as what we tell our hearts.

Working on all bodies together – the physical and energy bodies, as well as any others we may eventually discover – more easily brings body and Earth into alignment. Each feeds the other. Everything connects. How healthy we are is a result of how we choose to live our lives on every level. Even Dr. Carey Reams, who brought the soil-health link to the forefront said, "We don't live off the food we eat. We live off the energy of the food we eat. We live off the life in what's consumed."[415] How do we sustain the health and healing of our bodies and the planet? Take heart.

"The heart has reasons that reason cannot know."

~Blaise Pascal, French philosopher, inventor

Love Lessons

In his book *The Power of Now: A Guide to Spiritual Enlightenment*, Eckhart Tolle writes, "Love is not selective, just as the light of the sun is not selective. It does not make one person special. It is not exclusive. Exclusivity is not the love of God but the 'love' of ego. However, the intensity with which true love is felt can vary. There may be one person who reflects your love back to you more clearly and more intensely than others, and if that person feels the same toward you, it can be said that you are in a love relationship with him or her. The bond that connects you with that person is the same bond that connects you with the person sitting next to you on a bus, or with a bird, a tree, a flower. Only the degree of intensity with which it is felt differs."

Of all the reasons for creating the body, the most obvious one is to learn about love in its many forms. The challenge is working through the ego, the filter which shows us we always have the freedom to choose. We can choose to open our hearts or not. We can choose to stay where we are or move forward. Moving forward becomes a choice of opening the mind to the heart so the ego can be freed. It is a give-and-take between the heart and the head. Love is the question and the answer. To love and appreciate who we are brings draws to us the same love and appreciation in others. Relationships come into balance. Health comes into balance. The planet comes into balance.

Love is at the heart of all things. Love is consciousness. Love is light. Love is wisdom. Love is beauty. Love is awareness. Love is truth. Love is energy. Love is purity of spirit. You are thus energy without limit, beyond time and space, with no beginning and no end. Love can never be destroyed, only transformed into different states of itSelf. Love is never more or never less, it simply IS. Love is an IS-ness, a state of absoluteness that we bring to the world through the center of our physical being, and it is said to enter through the gate of the ego if the ego is open to receive it.

Love is not a constant state of bliss. Love knows and respects its opposite. But love requires opening up to the awareness that there is good in everything and everyone, and allowing that good energy to flow through amidst the chaos and distraction you perceive. If you can quiet the ego and watch your experiences as an observer, without getting stuck in those experiences, the ego's gate opens. And the heart opens to love. Observe your thoughts and with the heart direct them where you want them to go. When you see the your thoughts take shape in your reality, you know the universe has noticed you in the form of something you've noticed. Manifestation happens when words and actions align with truth. It happens in favor of the highest good. Simply say, "Thank you, universe! Looking forward to the next signs!"

Through love we become aware that we are being pulled toward something that is nameless. It may be a memory, or a longing from deep within. We sense it when we watch a play or a movie where love is lost or taken away. We feel a deep inexplicable emptiness. The solution is to go inside yourself, ground yourself, connect to your Self, and simply ask that love fill the space. You can also pick up some rose quartz, known as the stone of universal love. This crystal, when worn as jewelry or in your pocket or tucked in your pillowcase, offers a gentle, soft, up-lifting sensation. It enhances inner peace, self-worth, and love in all its forms. Washing your face in water charged by rose quartz is known to rejuvenate the skin. When you open your heart, other doors open. You experience a sense of being filled up to overflowing that cannot be experienced through the physical senses. It is a sense of the eventual return to the pure love.

Love Yourself

The universe is powered by love and through love. Love is the ultimate antidote for all suffering. No matter what insecurity we allow to consume our lives or what we think we need to fix about ourselves, it is our ability to love ourselves completely, including our flaws, which ultimately leads to true healing and transformation. This idea cannot be overstated.

Finding love for ourselves is not always easy. In life, we create walls around our hearts to protect them. We eat comfort food to fortify those walls and hide ourselves under the extra weight. We cover up with make-up to make ourselves pretty to others. In order to clear the walls and fortifications and reveal our true beauty, we need to clear trapped emotions and forgive ourselves. In order to clear the heart chakra, it may be helpful to first clear the first three. Most Americans are ungrounded in the first chakra, meaning the root chakra is blocked. This chakra at the based of the spine acts as a pump to help energy rise and flow. It represents connection to family and is the base of your emotional and mental center. A weak root chakra represents a lack of security, safety, and trust. It can be a lifelong process to clear this chakra or it can be instantaneous. It is completely individual and unique.

The solution to clearing chakras is found in love. When we love who we are, we create a place where specific change happens. Any discordant issue related to health, relationships, or career that shows up in our lives is an opportunity for us to deepen our capacity to bring love, give love, receive love, and accept love.

When you don't know the answers, defer to the heart. The heart knows. Always look internally for something beyond yourself and just out of reach. The only thing that fills the emptiness, whether from a feeling of sadness to a feeling of being pushed beyond limits, is the love that is found in the heart – your heart.

Heartbreak is not the end of any story. You are not bound to the ego's idea of love, a conditional love, which serves to bind and restrict. A marriage license does not contain the key to love just as a contract with the state is not a prerequisite to joining hearts. Sadly, couples often commit themselves to a license to love at the expense of being an expression of love. In administrative law, any license changes an inherent right into a privilege that can be taken away.

The unlegislated truth is that we are free to love whomever we choose, without conditions, from the privacy of our own hearts. This kind of love is beyond physical. It is not about sex. This is soul love. In this way, loving others we perceive to be inaccessible can be just as fulfilling as committing to one person alone. There are no restrictions whatsoever to love anyone, anywhere, at anytime, unconditionally. The heart's capacity for unconditional love is limitless, the gift that keeps on giving. No matter how many divergent or parallel paths we each walk, all roads on the spiritual path lead to love. The rest is just stuff.

The more we cultivate love, the more love we grow. Loving another's heart is loving their soul. We love their essence instead of the role they play in this life. Ram Dass, in his short film, "Love Serve Remember" said, "When you see someone's soul and notice their brilliance, they see you witnessing their brilliance and your spiritual heart radiates, giving them a feeling of what their spiritual heart is. Then, soul to soul, you rejoice in connection with soul."

A soul connection radiates love, truth, and peace beyond the linear confines of perception. When couples stay together "for the children" or for an image but without love, they are not living in truth or peace. The idea that there is never a good time to make a change or the belief that sticking it out is easier, actually sets the foundation that is often repeated in each successive generation. It is instructive that the bonds of marriage can and do create relationships where people feel powerless. Negative emotions manifest in the physical body to cause further damage.

However, it is only our perception that foundations and institutions are set in stone. In this era of dynamically shifting family structures, there are now many options that define a family. The once common nuclear family has morphed into equally shared parenting, the single-parent family, the step-family, the blended family, the childless family, the grandparent family, the extended family, and other variations. There is no limit to how families can transform themselves in healthy ways for the greatest good. The D-word need not reflect a sitcom or TV drama. Families can write, direct, and create their own story of reformation with love, where peace and balance are maintained.

> *"To forgive is to set a prisoner free and discover that the prisoner was you."*
>
> ~*Lewis B. Smedes, theologian*

Forgive Others

When you choose to forgive others who have hurt you, you gain back your power and your freedom. Whatever you perceive they did to you, realize that they were also doing it to themselves. Just as the transgression wasn't your fault it also wasn't theirs. Their choices reflected their own lack from their own wounds, from their own perspectives. Stories of abuse, whether physical or verbal, do not happen overnight. They come from a history of abuse, repeating energetic patterns that flow through generations. Society has taught us to demonize those who abuse without recognizing that the abuser has also suffered abuse. If it takes a village to raise a family, then where is the village when it comes to healing the abuse of the village?

What we give ourselves is what we get back. There is always a balance. If we don't have the capacity to forgive ourselves, the cycle of pain, resentment, and hate continues. If we don't have the ability receive love, we end up becoming martyrs, draining ourselves for the good of others. We must be able to forgive and receive for ourselves foremost. Only then can we give to others without losing ourselves. Giving and receiving needs to happen first from within before it can be shared from without. That perfect mate is ready to come walking through your door as soon as you release the battle wounds of past relationships.

Today's society raises families without an emphasis on community and raises whole communities without a sense of family. We are creating environments where people feel alone and empty, without connection or conviction. We are raising children who don't know the spirit of Self, the spirit of family, the spirit of community, or universal spirit.

The "zombie culture" of our youth is playing out in an epidemic of addiction to a designer drug from Russia called Krokodil, made from gasoline, lighter fluid, and codeine. The etiology of this drug kills the body from the inside-out, eating away at the flesh until only bone is visible. Disconnected from Self, this condition is a sign of the times, a reflection of the body and mind slowly disappearing because the spirit is being ignored.

"When you hold resentment toward another, you are bound to that person or condition by an emotional link that is stronger than steel. Forgiveness is the only way to dissolve that link and get free."

~Dr. William A. Tiller

Forgive Yourself

Only when we can forgive ourselves to accept all aspects of who we are can we heal in an authentic way. How do we forgive ourselves? The best way may be to have a conversation with your inner child who is always with you. See yourself as the mini-you looking up to greater-you and speak to her or him as you would a child. Remind your little self that what others have said about you is none of your business. It might read something like this:

Dear Little Self,

You are not your body. You are not your thoughts. And you are not what people have said you are. You are pure undeniable love. As long as you believed their words, they kept coming to you as mirrors to show you your shadows. Instead of turning away from their words, you chose to wear them as a suit of armor to protect yourself. Under all that armor, you couldn't see the light of your heart.

We are reflections of each other, you and me. I forgive you for holding onto those negative thoughts for so long and making yourself so small because you didn't know then what I know now. It is safe to take off the armor. I won't let any harm come to you.

You are beautiful and wise and loving and powerful. Your power comes from your spirit that cannot be bothered with thoughts or words. It is a place as vast as the universe with no space, time, depth, or physical sensation. It is beyond the senses. Your power is a river of love that flows through you, endless, full and peaceful.

What you didn't know is that you can take this river with you wherever you go. Stay in the flow and you will find whatever you need. In the silence of this river is where you find your true, perfect Self. You didn't see it before because your hands were too small to hold the mirror just right. Hold the mirror up. See that you are whole and complete and connected to everything and everyone. All you need is you.

Love always,
Higher Self

P.S. You weren't bossy. You have leadership skills. ☺

To love others we must first love ourselves and forgive ourselves. The emptiness or fullness in your self is a magnet that attracts others with the same lack, or richness, in their lives. When you serve others, you serve yourself, and vise versa. It is important to acknowledge and let go of any hurt, or lack, or animosity you still hold. It is perhaps the most important thing you can do to heal yourself because forgiveness is the greatest act of self-love.

Kim Phuc Phan Thi is now grown up. But she was once a girl who experienced the brutality of war. The date was June 8, 1972. The scene was a group of children fleeing the devastation created by a nuclear bomb dropped in South Vietnam by a pilot who mistook a group of civilians leaving the temple for enemy troops. The infamous black-and-white photograph won the Pulitzer Prize and was chosen as the World Press photo of Year in 1972, serving as a symbol of inhumanity and immorality. On December 28, 2009, National Public Radio broadcast her spoken essay "The Long Road to Forgiveness:"

"Forgiveness made me free from hatred. I still have many scars on my body and severe pain most days but my heart is cleansed. Napalm is very powerful, but faith, forgiveness, and love are much more powerful. We would not have war at all if everyone could learn how to live with true love, hope, and forgiveness."

With forgiveness, we connect to love and become compassionate toward ourselves and others. We see ourselves as part of the greater community. We find common ground to know we all just want to be loved. We see that we all come from the same place, all within the same presence of oneness. When the ego falls away, there is compassion and forgiveness. We can all entrain to the consciousness that lies within and realize that at our core we are all the same.

Forgive yourself for holding on to the pain for so long. Forgive yourself for infringing on others' energy. Let go of the ego, the hoarder of past judgments and resentments. Clear the path and move forward. It is never too late. There have been no wrong turns. Every up and down to this moment has been part of your life's path. By forgiving yourself as you forgive others, you offer two gifts to the universe, one for their healing, and one for yours.

Chapter Twenty-One

HEALING THE PLANET

She has a heartbeat. She breathes. She gives birth, she grows, she dies, and she is reborn with each cycle of the seasons. She has

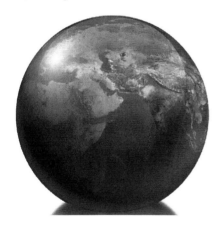

intelligence. Her name is Gaia, the great mother/goddess of all. According to ancient Greek religion, she is Earth personified. Gaia Theory suggests Gaia is a self-regulating complex biosystem where all lifeforms are considered part of one single living planet with the goal of sustaining optimal conditions for all life.

Working with the sun and the entire solar system, Mother Earth maintains all systems go. She cycles and recycles so that nothing is wasted. Just as living beings breathe out carbon dioxide, which is cycled through plants and returned as oxygen, we get what we give. Our interactions in Nature boomerang back to us. Nurturing and care results in health for all. Recklessness and negligence produces uncontrolled releases of toxic waste into our water, land, air, and our cells.

There is a deep consciousness that binds all life on the planet together. The 1979 documentary *The Secret Life of Plants* reveals the physical, emotional, and spiritual interactions between plants and humans.[416] Plants have intelligence despite their lack of a physical brain and nervous system. As depicted by Cleve Backster's plant experiments using the human polygraph test, plants actively engage in their environment. They cooperate with each other, respond to predators nurture their young, and can even wage war. They communicate and respond to our presence, as perceived when the electrical output of plants is translated into sound through computer modulation.[417]

"Every tree, every plant has a spirit. People may say that a plant has no mind. I tell them that a plant is alive and conscious. A plant may not talk, but there is a spirit in it that is conscious, that sees everything, which is the soul of the plant, its essence, what makes it alive."

~Pablo Amaringo, Peruvian artist and shaman

The series of destructive events happening around the planet have reached a climax if measured solely by the ever-growing and frustrated voices of protest around the world. People are coming together to herald a wake-up call to the most critical issues of the day – the genetic manipulation and control of the food supply by a few corporations, the transfer of wealth to large corporate entities, and the restriction of personal freedoms by federal laws that have turned inherent rights into privileges that can be taken away.

Peaceful demonstrations and marches not only signal a shift in the status quo, they also reflect the Earth's immune system activating her power to heal herself. All over the world a restless energy is being unleashed in favor of the our natural rights to life, liberty, and the pursuit of happiness, the ideals reflected in America's Declaration of Independence written in 1776:

When in the Course of human events, it becomes necessary for one people to dissolve the political bands which have connected them with another, and to assume among the powers of the earth, the separate and equal station to which the Laws of Nature and of Nature's God entitle them, a decent respect to the opinions of mankind requires that they should declare the causes which impel them to the separation....That whenever any Form of Government becomes destructive of these ends, it is the right of the People to alter or to abolish it, and to institute new Government, laying its foundation on such principles, and organizing its powers in such form, as to them shall seem most likely to effect their Safety and Happiness... it is their right, it is their duty, to throw off such Government, and to provide new Guards for their future security.

Today's urgency revolves around the need for truth, sustainability, unity, equality, health, and healing for all life on the planet. No government or institution or scientism can stand in the way of the will of the people or the will of the planet to achieving the greatest good for all life. Such is the law of Nature.

Just as societies grow from within, they also fall from within. Evidence is showing that old belief systems are crumbling as whole nations choose to reject what no longer serves them. Genetically modified seeds and foods are being burned, banned, or refused entry across foreign borders. Native seeds are being saved. Our very cells are speaking out against denatured foods through the symptoms of disease, demanding that we return to the Earth for healing. Mother Earth is not passive in self-healing as she purges and cleanses with increased severity and frequency through natural disasters such as earthquakes, hurricanes, and sinkholes.

"I predict future happiness for Americans if they can prevent the government from wasting the labors of the people under the pretense of taking care of them."

~Thomas Jefferson, author "Declaration of Independence"

The myths of "improving Nature" with the genetically modified organism are being exposed as false as we open to truth and become willing to think independently. Contrary to manufacturer claims, GMO "Franken-crops" are less productive,[418] with fewer yields.[419] They are more resistant to pesticides, and create superbugs,[420] and

225

super-weeds.[421] They have caused substantial increases in pesticide use.[422] Studies continue to show that conventional plant breeding – not genetic engineering – is responsible for higher yields in crops.[423] What else should we expect from a knock-off, anyway?

GMO residues leach into the water supply to damage aquatic life and all who drink it and up to seventeen percent of pathogens survive wastewater treatment due to the high levels of antibiotics and anti-bacterial ingredients (e.g., Triclosan®) found there.[424] Carried by the wind, GMO seeds eliminate biodiversity through genetic drift, to con-taminate and sterilize native plants. Genetic drift creates monocul-tures of seed crops, depleting the soil of minerals and life. GMO seed companies threaten the control of the global seed supply through a monopoly and private patents.[425]

The promise of GMO foods to feed the world has only served to starve it since the majority of GMO crops are grown to feed livestock, not humans. The decline in biodiversity also results from pollination by bees that transfer GMO pollen to native plant species, and has directly led to the collapse of bee populations around the world due to toxic neonicotinoids in the pesticides.[426] [427]GMO technology destroys the same metabolic pathways of bees, plants, and that of our own gut bacteria.[428]

Cloning human embryos for "therapeutic purposes" was made le-gal in England in 2001.[429] Next in the GMO pipeline are human genes into the foods we eat – cannibalism.[430] The group that brought us Aspartame and Round Up are the same ones that introduced rBGH in milk, petroleum-based fertilizers, Dioxin, Agent Orange, the atomic bomb, and nuclear waste.

Like Big Pharma, Big Ag GMO corporations grant themselves all the rights of "personhood" then exempt themselves from liability or accountability through legislation.[431] They exploit farmers through contracts that turn farmers into indentured servants, requiring them to purchase patented seeds annually, as well as expensive pesticides and energy-intensive heavy equipment needed to apply them. Since 1997, over 200,000 farmers in India, alone, have committed suicide from the pressure of high debts they were unable to pay off for the first time in their family's history.[432]

In our drive to create complex societies, we have overlooked the simple truth that it is our Earth that sustains us. That which we do to the Earth we do to ourselves. In our surrender of personal power, we allow farm policy to create monocultures of our food, medical policy to create monocultures of our bodies, educational policy to create monocultures of our minds, and warring policy to create monocultures of whole nations. One system reflects all systems.

We carry this loss of power into our personal lives. We suppress physical symptoms with drugs, repress emotions with excuses, and deny our wisdom in favor of others.' We plead ignorance and frustration because there are just too many distractions from science and technology in its details, its catalog of definitions, its speed and agility, and its delivery systems. As long as the blinders remain fixed we allow systems to control us and determine the outcomes.

As long as we compartmentalize the body and build monuments to Heart Center or the Digestive Center or the Cancer Center, we fail to see the whole person. For the last hundred years, the American Cancer Society, ever in search of "the cure," has only documented increases in cancer death rates. According to the latest meta-analysis on breast screening published in the November 2012 *New England Journal of Medicine*, over the past thirty years, 1.3 million American women were wrongly diagnosed and treated for breast 'cancers' they never had.

"Not one cell in your body is made from a drug."

~Andrew W. Saul, Doctor Yourself Newsletter (April, 2006)

Resistance is Futile

The tragedy that cancer death rates have not improved, but only increased over time can be tied to the tools of industrial medicine (surgery, irradiation, chemotherapy, synthetic drugs) that have resisted change for over fifty years.

Perhaps the poor prognosis is due to flawed drug study designs that do not conduct placebo (no-treatment) controlled, double blind studies against new toxic drugs (i.e., chemotherapy) due to the ethics excuse that all participants should receive treatment.[433] Or perhaps, the placebo effect is really just a label for the body's natural healing process. Dr. Peter Gotzsche, MD, professor and director of The Nordic Cochrane Centre in Copenhagen, Denmark says, "In a study where one group gets an SSRI and the other a placebo, you can't claim anything on the efficacy of the placebo. It's definitely not 50%. And why not? Because if you had a third group which received no treatment, not even a placebo, about half would recover by themselves! That means that it's not placebo effect: It's the spontaneous healing process of the illness- which is primarily why 50% feel better on the placebo."[434] Perhaps cancer rates have only increased because alternative approaches using nutrition-based controls are systematically undermined and are set up to fail based on the "bias, indifference and ...incompetence" of the system.[435]

The system cherry-picks information and chooses to ignore research that shows how the most prevalent herbicide in the western diet, GMO glyphosate is a xeno-estrogen that promotes all forms of cancer, especially estrogen-dependent (breast) cancer cell growth at levels in parts per trillion.[436] This knowledge has been suppressed for too long, yet it is deeply relevant to all who eat food for sustenance. In trusting the system, we are distracted with "Race for the Cure®" instead of focusing on the cause.

We allow corporations to alter and patent Nature for profit while suppressing natural alternatives for all. In our apathy and sedation we have denied ourselves full access to knowledge and truth and disconnected from our rightful inheritance to all the Earth provides. Nature is not patentable. Nor does the Earth discriminate against who can and cannot partake of its offerings. So why do we allow it? We belong to the Earth as much as the Earth belongs to all of us.

As Tiller observed, "Science cannot give you truth. All it can determine is internal self-consistency" based on data within the confines of time and distance. Everything else must be rejected. Natural phenomena – emotion, mind, spirit, intention, love, consciousness – are not valid in the science paradigm. In a White Paper on the mind-body energy system, William Tiller argues that the placebo event in the doctor-patient relationship is not an inert entity of the system "but rather is elevated to the state of a dynamic 'player' via quantum entanglement with all the other 'players.'"[437] The mind cannot be overlooked in outcomes without denying who we are. We must understand that if we are to evolve our beingness we must acknowledge our electromagnetic selves and how all energetic modalities – from acupuncture to homeopathy to naturopathy to energy medicine – work directly on the inner Self, then indirectly on the physical self.

The Return to Nature

In this moment in time, we have reached a precipice as a species. It has been our nature to edit Nature as we see it. As always, the answer to recovering our balance – before we fall over the edge – is to return to Nature in its pure state.

In his book *Children of Dune*, Frank Herbert writes:

> A sophisticated human can become primitive. What this really means is that the human's way of life changes. Old values change, become linked to the landscape with its plants and animals. This new existence requires a working knowledge of those multiples and cross-linked events usually referred to as nature. It requires a measure of respect for the inertial power within such natural systems. When a human gains this working knowledge and respect, that is called "being primitive."

The spirit is our ever-patient guide, always ready and willing to help heal the break and bring us back into alignment. Spirit has never been suppressed or confined by any construct including systems, time-space, or a body for that matter. Our individual spirit naturally leads us to discover individual truth. We only need to allow it to guide us.

The many challenges we face represent opportunities for all of us on our planet. We must see them as symptoms of the human condition. We are each responsible for our health as well as the health and well-being of the planet. Being responsible means coming into one's power and recognizing that this power ripples out to affect the collective. Acting on behalf of the Earth, not only can we reverse the putrification we see around us, we can prevent new infections.

The New World Disorder

The phrase "the new world order" has been uttered by many-a-world leader over the decades as a plan for how duality reality will continue to unfold in world affairs. But plans change. People wake up. Welcome to the Information Age. Thanks to instant mass communication through the internet, the world is experiencing an unprecedented and accelerated universal awakening of consciousness. Goodbye to the Germ Theory. Humankind is going Viral. The *many* are now making an impact in trends of thought on a massive scale.

"Persistent and highly motivated populist resistance of politically awakened and historically resentful peoples to external control has proven to be increasingly difficult to suppress."[314]

~ *Zbigniew Brzezinski, Trilateral Commission Co-founder*

The dramas unfolding are not merely physical in nature. They are energetic. Blatant and excessive control and power grabs by authorities represent acts of desperation by an elite who are fast losing their grip. Authority only perceives it has power over others as long as the People believe themselves to be oppressed. Enslavement in society does not come through laws and statutes. It comes through psychological manipulation so that consciousness creates such a reality. Those within the system often do not perceive that they are imprisoned because they do not realize there is something outside of where they exist.

"I freed a thousand slaves. I could have freed a thousand more if only they knew they were slaves."

~ *Harriet Tubman, Underground Railroad conductor.*

When propagandists and apologists bang the drums of fear in light of growing personal power, it fully reflects systems of external control on the verge of collapse. The energies playing out today are symptoms of change as natural as a volcanic eruption or a bud pushing through the soil. Any birthing process includes a level of distress as new life emerges. As our world transforms to a balanced state, structures that are unsustainable – whether economic, medicinal, environmental, political, or personal – will collapse of their own low-vibrational weight. The demise of structures is not to be feared. It is a natural consequence of irrelevancy. Out with the old and in with the new.

Energies that do not align with truth, justice, and love will naturally be cleansed and removed, just as the human body cleanses itself when faced with the introduction of a toxin to its terrain. This is expressed in Chaos Theory which applies to non-linear system and states that when systems appear to spiral out of control a dramatic shift takes place that takes reality to a new, higher dynamic, a more evolved state of being. We only need to embody the perception that reality does not happen to us. We make it happen.

The process of detoxification whether in our internal or external environments is not good or bad, light or dark. It is not about one group labeled entitled and another labeled paranoid. It just IS. It is Nature in its natural state, working to find balance, as Nature is designed to do. Deepak Chopra says, "All great changes are preceded by chaos." At this time in our evolution we are merely experiencing the storm before the calm.

Empower and Revalue

According to the Mayans as well as other indigenous cultures, we have just completed a great cycle of approximately 25,000 years and also a grand cycle of approximately 125,000 years. Earth is moving across the Galactic equator which offers a window of alignment with that central energy. If time appears to be speeding up, it might be reflective of nearing that zero point of no-time where past, present, and future converge.

As individuals who mirror greater universal evolutionary changes, we must make the most of this opportunity to manifest what serves us all for the highest good. In this moment of no-time we can become grounded human beings, and separate from the emotional energy of this new birth. The simple act of walking barefoot in the grass and getting your hands dirty by working with the Earth will bring a deep sense of belonging.

It is time to take off the armor worn out during the initial battles. It has brought us to this point in time and served us well. Now is the time to open our hearts to our innate gifts and become more conscious. We can use our voices for peace and our bodies to create a world that empowers each of us.

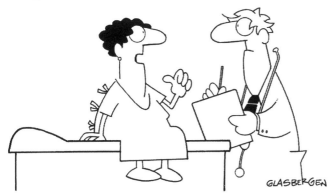

"You have to learn about thousands of diseases, but I only have to focus on fixing what's wrong with ME! Now which one of us do you think is the expert?"

Now is place to transcend our differences, to find balance, and to work as one. We are all in this together.

We are reminded that our reality is made up of atoms that are mostly empty space. Consisting mostly of bacteria, we see that we are only as healthy as our smallest inhabitants. Anything is possible when you realize who you truly are. You are your own expert.

Food

We can each vote with our fork, grow our own food in community gardens or in our own yards, for a reliable and safe domestic food supply. We can join a local Food Swap Network.[438] We can support local, small farmers to keep the soil nourished and keep economies local. We can create private food buying clubs and healthcare memberships that are completely self-sufficient and outside the jurisdiction of the system.

Money

We can opt out of the corrupt, monopolized, debt-based monetary system that keeps people dependent and powerless. Instead, we can raise and pool our money through "crowd funding," bypassing the banks that create fiat money out of thin air. We can build our own decentralized banking system bartering services using our gifts.

The debt-based monetary system is a reflection of our perceived lack of value based on a belief system that keeps us separate from everything. We can no more spend ourselves out of debt than secure inherent freedoms by allowing government to control us. Broken into its roots, *govern* (to control or regulate) and *ment* (the action or state of) is the act of controlling others. How does one entity protect the freedoms of an individual through control?

Instead, we can build our own decentralized banking system by bartering services using our gifts. Timebanking is a system where the medium exchanged is time and energy. Everyone's time is valued equally where one hour of service earns one credit-hour. Timebanking builds community by valuing the contributions of all, matching unused resources with unmet needs. In such a regional collaboration, members can earn time credits by contributing skilled services or skill building in any creative capacity. Anyone who has earned can spend. As members offer their time, skills, and energy, they create a community "bank" of skills on which others can draw.[439]

"When freedom is outlawed only outlaws will be free."

~Author Unknown

We empower ourselves when we come together and see ourselves as one heart and one mind working for the greatest good. There is no price on our heads. We are priceless. True originals. Masterpieces. Yet we are the only species that pays to live on Earth. We only need to accept the truth that I AM the value. Only then will false symbols (e.g., fiat paper currency) fall away for good.

After all, it has always been us who holds the real value, not any politician, bank, currency, or government bond. Government authorities know well our true worth. Each of us collectively comprises the total wealth of our country. Resources may be considered assets, but without our energy, our country is worthless, our economy baseless. A farmer cultivates the soil, plants the seeds, and harvests the bounty with his hands and his skill. Vegetables must be dug up and bagged before they are available to buy and eat. The soil without this effort is just dirt. Touching the Earth has fringe benefits. It literally connects us to our roots and our true value. When we eat sprouts (germinating seeds of life) full of chi, we build our own chi.

"In nature's economy the currency is not money it is life."

~Vandana Shiva, author, environmental activist

Government

We become "game changers" when using words that reflect our full worth. We can say no to contradictions of common sense and act on them. We can claim our rights, regain our power, and nullify laws that do not serve the highest good. We can act under the Precautionary Principle by supporting a moratorium on denatured seed technologies, and at the same time hold government accountable for damage that continues in our name.

Building a free system is accomplished not through signing petitions that agencies ignore. Petitioning government is nothing more than asking for permission (i.e. begging). All begging is a form of consent. If we do not consent to GMO food then the strongest action we can take is to stop eating it. GMO company employees don't eat their own food, so why should we? Boycotting GMO food – 90 percent of processed foods – is the most efficient way to hit them where it hurts; the bottom line.

We are our environment, our government, and our economy. Natural rights are our birthright and can neither be given away nor denied by any government or court. Judges nearly file opinions. It is the court's job to uphold rights.

> "The rights of the individual are not derived from governmental agencies, either municipal, state or federal, or even from the Constitution. They exist inherently in every man, by endowment of the Creator, and are merely reaffirmed in the Constitution, and restricted only to the extent that they have been voluntarily surrendered by the citizenship to the agencies of government. The people's rights are not derived from the government, but the government's authority comes from the people. The Constitution but states again these rights already existing, and when legislative encroachment by the nation, state, or municipality invade these original and permanent rights, it is the duty of the courts to so declare, and to afford the necessary relief. The fewer restrictions that surround the individual liberties of the citizen, except those for the preservation of the public health, safety, and morals, the more contented the people and the more successful the democracy." (City of Dallas v. Mitchell, 245 S.W. 944, 945-46, Tex.Civ.App. – Dallas (1922).

We are a self-organizing species that can come together as equals who live in harmony and autonomy under rules without rulers. Authority figures will automatically label such a concept as anarchy and demonize those who promote it in order to maintain control. But that is their definition of a structure promoting personal freedom in a voluntary-based system.[440] To create such freedom it will take each of us to accept personal responsibility for all of our actions. And self-control. Peaceful rule is possible if we follow three simple rules: 1) Follow your passion and respect others to do the same, 2) Do no harm, and 3)

There are no other rules. To live free is to be free. Once a majority of us revalue ourselves, we raise the bar for all. Mountains move.

When we build community with our neighbors we eliminate the need for representative government. As Einstein once said, "No problem can be solved from the same level of consciousness that created it." When we reject the perceptions of fear, anxiety, rage, and guilt, we naturally make room to perceive forgiveness, joy, peace, and love. We move in a new direction to create a new reality on Earth. When we live out our gifts and live in harmony with the planet we live in our true essence. We become and unfold to our natural state. We become less dense. As we merge our darker aspects with our light we transform through the heart, the center of our being and the center of the universe. We see our own transformation reflect in our reality because reality reflects where we are right now. What happens within manifests without. What we do in our inner spiritual world feeds that transformational power. We only need to be aware of our potential.

Accessing our true potential means that we are self-assured in our creative capacities. Being self-assured relates to our emotions. It's psychological, not logical. We must silence the logical brain from its propensity to analyze every detail of existence and simply work to change our assumptions. The law of attraction mirrors the law of assumptions.[441] When we open to the power of imagination, we guide our emotions in a positive direction. To create the outcome we want we must be in the moment, using the right tense. We say, "I am..." instead of "I will be..." or I am going to be..." We must use our creative gifts.

"You are very powerful, provided you know how powerful you are."

~Yogi Bhajan

We have always had access, and power to change our reality, we have only forgotten. Our capacity to remember is found by reconnecting to Nature. As part of Nature our answers are stored in our spiritual hard drive as love and in our universal hard drive as water. All life on Earth comes back to basic universal elements, to water and oxygen. Seventy percent of the Earth's surface is covered by water, similar to the percentage of water found in the human body. We have the potential to create peace or a cleaner planet simply by remembering that we are the Holy Grail containing all the tools we need.

Water, The Universal Communicator

Japanese researcher Masaro Emoto's controversial water experiments showed how the properties of water and the power of intention have the potential to restructure polluted water to its pure state at the subatomic level. In exposing water to words (including prayer), sounds, and intentions, Emoto tested the theory that the memory of water is another fractal of consciousness with the power to restructure itself.[442] Scientists over the world are showing that water may have the ability to communicate instantaneously.[443] In a 2008 in Russia, Emoto conducted a ceremonial blessing of Lake Baikal, the world's deepest freshwater lake. Using an electrophotonic camera, sensors measured changes of capacitance of several elements – water, earth, plant, and air. The data showed distinct differences at various stages of the ceremony.[444]

Current restructuring water systems allow anyone to improve the quality of their water from their home and wherever they go. These technologies can be used reclaim wastewater as well as polluted lake ecosystems. The options are endless, including bacteria to clean water[445] or a simple bed of algae, using sunlight as a fuel source.[446] Sound frequencies of the sun – 124 Hz – and of music – 528 Hz – are also known to harmonize water and affect the body.[447] Tests conducted using the sound of the sun – using a electrophotonic camera to monitor the human bioenergy field from a person's fingertips – showed increases in energy patterns radiating from that person's heart. Being exposed the sound of a solar flare for one minute activated the human heart.

Many critics will criticize the new technologies and claim Emoto's experiments are not reproducible. It is important to be open to news ways of thinking if anything is to change. Be aware that orthodox science operates within self-imposed limits. Remember, too, the Observer Effect is always in play – subatomic particles behave in the way people think. You find what you look for.

Because everything is energy, everything is alive. Water is alive as much as plants are alive as much as we are alive. The information contained in water may reflect the information of the Akashic records.[449] After all, consciousness and matter are intrinsically linked.

Each of us by our very nature has the potential to access this energy. Thanks to Emoto's work, the possibilities are endless in our ability to reclaim the oceans from pollution, the land from nuclear contamination, and the body from disease. When each of us join hearts and minds the effect of one is multiplied exponentially. The square root of one percent of the world's populations, a mere 7,000 people, can change anything we wish to change as long as we focus our minds together with heartfelt intention. Change never happens in the future. Change happens here and now, within each of us, when we all work together.

Remember, the capacity to accept change without fear is found through love. Love is the power that underlies everything. Everything is either love or a cry for love. Love is the means and the end. We come from love, are born into love, grow in love, and we return to love. Love is all there is. Unconditional love is the essence of who we are as spirit beings. It is the life force. It is not romantic love. It simply asks that we accept others without judgment or expectations, no matter what they say or how they act, since they create their own stories for their own soul experiences. As each of us sees truth from our own perspective, we must recognize that each person sees truth through his own eyes based on his own beliefs.

"The world is changed by your example, not by your opinion."

~Paul Coelho, author

All energy is potential love if we choose to feel it. Though it may change form throughout life based on our perceptions, love never leaves. Nothing else matters. Not materialism. Not things. In reality there are only probabilities of interconnections. There are no objects, only relationships. Take up your power cord and pulse your unique energy over the Earth for the greatest good. Send love to the hearts of those who suffer and those who promote the suffering (they need it most). Realize your true value is all you.

Chapter Twenty-Two

THE POWER TO CHOOSE

"There are two primary choices in life; to accept conditions as they exist, or accept the responsibility for changing them."

~Denis Waitley

All the moments of your life have brought you to this one. You are here based on your beliefs, thoughts, and actions. No experience was wasted effort since each was a choice. The changes you make are always choices. Life is a series of choices. Own them and know that you are right where you need to be. All is well.

Spirit has led you on this healing journey to find your higher self. Your higher self wants you to know that you are a true gift and it is high time to start appreciating the gift that you are. Look in the mirror and tell yourself that you are awesomeness. Celebrate yourself. Be your own hero. Be a sense-ation because you are a sensory being. Allow your heart chakra to open wide. Appreciate who you are and know that who you are is enough. Live in each moment because every moment is a gift. That is why we call it the present. Each moment presents a new opportunity and another choice to make. Knowing that we have enough in each moment makes us feel abundant. It naturally shifts our energy vibration from scarcity to fulfillment.

We each hold the power to create angst or peace, disease or health. As beings who create from each moment, it becomes important to live in each moment. Only then do we become centered in our own awareness where truth is revealed. We allow our creative light to be expressed and shared.

Being in the moment means you have found the course of least resistance. The universe aligns in your favor. You become aware of the messages, the signs, and symbols that direct you on your path. New opportunities flow to you as you recognize your inner artist creates your life, the artist your soul created. And though your time in your body is limited, the soul never dies. So make the best use of your body while you have it.

We each hold the power to create angst or peace, disease or health. As beings who create from each moment, it becomes important to live in each moment. Only then do we become centered in our own awareness where truth is revealed. We allow our creative light to be expressed and shared.

By living truth in the moment we declare who we are, we create our life with purpose and conviction. We become the "I" of the storm of swirling opinions. We let go of past opinions and past judgments. We free ourselves to see all of us as one. The past is a memory and the future hasn't yet arrived, and never will. As Eckhart Tolle writes, "You are not the past, nor the future. You are the now." Likewise, the children are not the future. They are the present.

Like a tree, you are a channel of light connecting the Earth to the universe, grounded and open to higher dimensions. You need only open your branches and allow the light flow through you to positively affect others and your world. Sharing your gifts is the best way to do this. Finding your creative gifts and sharing them with others is why you are here.

Let your inner child come out to play and watch your life expand as you experience your world in a state of awe and gratitude. There is a path laid out for you and by you, but you always have free will, the freedom to make slight adjustments in each moment. Nothing is set in stone. You can choose to see fearful images, anger, greed, hate, separation, or destruction. Or you can choose to see beauty, goodness, love, unity, and abundance. Life presents the colors but it is how you choose to paint the image that determines the final creation. You are an original. Choose to be who you are.

Be Open and Be Grateful

Choose to be open to your awareness. Once you realize your relationships and your environment are a direct reflection of what you think and feel inside, you have accepted your power to change your entire outward experience. You realize you cannot blame others for your lot in life for at your core it was always you at the controls.

After being sick and tired of facing the same outcomes, spirit always offers the choice to be open-minded. This means being willing to learn, take risks, trust, and discover further truths that might not agree with past belief systems.

When you choose to be open-minded by letting go of patterns that hold you back, you shift your energy. When you align with your true gifts, and with your higher self. The universe conspires to bring you more of what you seek for your greatest good and for that of humanity.

"When we open our minds to anything and everything, anything and everything starts to reveal itself."

~Author Unknown

We are made up of both feminine and masculine energies, yin and yang. We are the perfection of pure spirit which manifests the body. As the spirit is perfect, so too is the body. In the body, each cell has a specialized function and works together to sustain the whole. The same is true for humanity in which we each play a role. Each of us is a thread in the fabric.

Nature is life in balance. To ignore Nature is to ignore who we are. When we live life disconnected from ourselves, we disconnect from others, as well as the planet. When we pollute our air and water, we hurt ourselves and all species.

Be grateful. We have everything now. We live in abundance everyday. We only have to realize it. However you describe it, abundance is not measurable. You cannot qualify it as "yes, but..." or quantify it as "yes, but more is better." Abundance is the sweetness of life and sweetness is not measurable. Eating a gallon of raw honey is just as sweet as tasting one finger full. Sweetness is sweetness.

Being grateful, like being present, takes practice. The more you do it, the more proficient you become. You hear a song on the radio and it speaks to you. It plays just for you. Be grateful for love in the form of music. You create a meal from locally grown food because you have access to foods of your choice. Be grateful for our "collective mother"

Earth who sustains all. You go to bed with a list of things still left to do. Be grateful for what you did accomplish. You wake up in the morning full of energy. Be grateful for new opportunities that present themselves in each moment. Be open and be grateful for the people present in your life and what they teach you about yourself, about what you can tolerate and what you cannot or should not. Be grateful for the ability to affect others by your smile and by the smiles that are returned to you.

"Gratitude paints little smiley faces on everything it touches."

~Richelle E. Goodrich, author

As we each become more aware of our presence and what we can create, we bring new experiences that lead to new opportunities for which to be grateful. The mind is stretched. The soul grows. Mind and soul can never revert back to their old dimensions – even if the body can. As the soul grows, so does all of humanity. Each generation sustains a higher level of consciousness than the one before. As human consciousness expands so does the consciousness of the planet. These ideas are expressed through many ancient religious texts including: "The Upanishads," The Bhagavad-Gita," and "The Kabbalah." The ultimate purpose of spirit is to bring matter back to pure light energy once again. This describes the evolution of the soul. Be grateful that you are a part of this creative process.

If you are grateful you are not fearful. Scarcity changes to joy and happiness. Our world is transformed. As our imaginations break free of old limits, we allow ourselves the freedom to think beyond what has already been, to create new paradigms. We can believe what our episenses tell us even if our physical senses fall short. Imagination is the key to greater awareness. As soul beings, we are ever evolving for the greatest good because we all come from the same home, and that home is inside us. When we see our nature reflecting in others around us then we have the wisdom to come together as one.

Our nature *is* Nature, and Nature aligns with truth. Living in truth means aligning our words with our actions. Understanding the congruency between truth and Nature represents a growing consciousness. A new way of seeing and being. Being clear who we are with our

THE POWER TO CHOOSE

words and actions brings us to that new consciousness. We haven't arrived late to this awareness because everything happens in the right time. We are meant to live and think freely even if the ego in its tunnel vision believes it is the master of its house.

Recognize fear for what it is. Fear is a choice. It is merely a belief that holds us back and tests us. We can transform that wave energy from potential to kinetic. Like arrows notched and drawn on the bow, we can propel ourselves into our true presence. The simple way to let go of fear is to be present and be grateful.

Bring It!

Where your attention goes, so goes your energy. What you look for you will find. If you focus your attention on the truth of all that you are, that is what you will naturally attract into your life. Like attracts like. In his book *The Moses Code*, author James Twyman writes about manifesting what you desire by bringing it through the soul. It is not about bringing in material wants (car, money, house) or even companions (kids, partners, pets) through the ego to puff it up. It is about bringing in your deepest yearning, passion, purpose, compassion, love, joy, and peace through the gifts you were born with. Through sharing your creative gifts you will also bring in whatever else is required for your needs (car, money, partners, kids).

The code is really your intention or declaration for what you choose to manifest by embodying the feeling of Oneness, and living in the now. You simply make it so, in the present tense. Using the breath, you say and feel what you choose to be, I AM Complete. I AM Healthy. I AM Peace. I AM the voice that comforts someone. I AM love here to make a difference for the greater good. And don't forget to say I AM grateful. Say them out loud. Then repeat. It is the repetition, like a mantra, that encodes this energy frequency into your cells to manifest your experiences, including the experience of full health and vitality.

Ride the Vibrational Wave of Consciousness

The universe always aligns to work in your favor without judgment. The potential for positive or negative outcomes is yours at every moment as reflected in the amplitude and depth of a wave. The excitement of your goals can be canceled by the doubt of your anxiety. The outcome is based on the frequencies of what you project from the inside. Recognize that what is missing is what you are not allowing to come in.

"If you surrender to the wind, you can ride it."

~Toni Morrison, poet

Indian yogi and guru, Paramahansa Yogananda lived in accordance with law of attraction at a very high level. He showed by example that we can put ourselves in a state of vibration that attracts what we need and that our potential is as great as we can imagine. If he lacked iron in his blood, Yogananda could attract iron to himself through his mental concept of the element iron. In this way, the frequency of the thought of iron manifested as a nutrient food source.

Though we may be far from Yogananda's abilities, we all have the capacity to practice riding the vibrational wave to see how it plays out in our lives. In order for it to play out as we want, we must believe it before we see it, not see it before we believe it. Trusting the process is key. We choose to ride the side of the wave we want to manifest. Simply be in the vibration of what we want – joy, love, enthusiasm, compassion – and watch it materialize. Manifesting our dreams is not only about dreaming. It requires acting on them. The challenge is to act no matter what the pressure or stressor from society, parents, peers, doctors, politicians, etc. Refuse to be defined by others.

When we are clear about what moves us, we magnetically draw people and situations that align with us who further propel us forward. We receive information at the right moment. We are each the student asking questions and the teacher providing insight to others. We assist each other by our very presence. When we collectively put our desires out to the universe as a declaration – then let it go – like a boomerang the answer will come back to us in dreams, people, and events. Pay attention to what is happening around you in your world and in the greater world. There is wisdom in every symbol and every word. The answer is on its way and it travels on the waves of consciousness.

"Don't dismiss the synchronicity of what is happening right now finding its way into your life at just this moment. There are no coincidences in the universe, only convergences of will, intent and experience."

~Neale Donald Walsch

Consciousness exists in all things. It is found within each cell, between cells, among groups of cells (tissues), in organ systems, in thoughts, between thoughts, in each of us, in groups of us, among each species on the planet, in the planet, between planets, and on and on. Consciousness is always spinning out in its creative expression through all life to understand itself.

Entrainment

As words, ideas, and experiences ripple out, they become part of the collective, expanding consciousness. As these resonant energies harmonize and flow outward in the web, we ultimately reach a tipping point that enables all minds to come together no matter where we are. This energetic phenomenon may have been described first by Dutch physicist Christian Huygens in the 1600s as *entrainment*, when two or more oscillating systems (e.g., metronomes mounted on a common board) naturally fall into synchrony.

Synchrony happens when a warm hand holding a cold lemonade glass warms the glass and cools the hand toward a happy medium. Energy adjusts between potential energy and kinetic energy to equalize two or more interacting systems to assume a more stable relationship. This natural rule applies universally over so many dynamics – thermal, kinetic, sonic, so why not in social structures like warring nations or human relationships?

The Hundreth Monkey

The expanding nature of consciousness was also observed by a group of scientists on the island of Koshima in Japan, who had been observing a group of monkeys for a period of thirty years in what became known as the Hundreth Monkey Phenomenon. In 1952, the scientists provided the monkeys with raw sweet potatoes dropped in the sand. Not finding sandy potatoes appealing, one 18-month old female washed the potato in a stream and taught this act to her mother. Soon other playmates followed and taught their mothers. Once a certain critical mass of monkeys (the exact number is unknown) attained this new awareness, suddenly all monkeys everywhere, on and off the island, knew the same skill. Monkey consciousness had forever shifted, revealing that such a change is communicated from mind to mind.[450]

While some may question the simplicity of this example, it well describes a tipping point that is reached in the biofield when the power of one individual aids in expanding consciousness for the whole web. The Hundreth Monkey Phenomenon describes an individual consciousness and a greater consciousness, a single mind and a one mind that connects us all. When we see that we are all connected to each other, we reach a place of entrainment. The ego will have done its job and can be laid to rest. The distractions and differences that take away our energy, the differences between people we perceive with our eyes, will fall away like layers of an onion.

This unseen unified whole has been expressed since the beginning of recorded time by all religions of the world. When Jesus said, "The Kingdom of God is within you," he lived this kingdom as unconditional love, joy, and peace of mind. This kingdom is not found in Vatican City guarded by men adorned in red robes. They do not hold the golden key because nothing is locked. Besides, there is no "us" and "them." The kingdom is Source and it is not outside of us. Source is us.

> *"Humanity is being guided to purer and deeper realms of consciousness beyond our current perception wherein we realize and rediscover deepened abilities we've been taught to believe couldn't possibly exist."*
>
> *~Wes Annac blog*

Living from this perspective, we as artists are capable of being and becoming anything we choose to be. We are creative expressions of Oneness and have the ability to create peace and heal ourselves as soon as we decide to do so. Nothing is beyond us. Nothing has power over us. Everything is within our reach. We only need to go inside and stand in our power. Knowing who we are is our connection to Source. We nurture this connection by caring for the soul like we care for the body, the temple of the soul. We nurture the body by cultivating and replenishing the soil, and by eating unadulterated foods directly from the Earth.

Our food, like us, is more than meets the eye. Each plant contains its own wisdom and resonates in wholeness at its true frequency, finding balance with its own surroundings. Raising our own food ensures that we put pure, clean energy into our bodies. It is not the food itself but the energy of the food that sustains the body, mind, and spirit. We naturally expand our consciousness and the consciousness of the Earth when we put our individual energy into the soil where we live.

As we ground ourselves, we access our higher selves and exchange this energy with others and with our environment to entrain and come into balance. Being in the flow of consciousness brings freedom, self-expression, collaboration of minds, creativity and connection, all which help merge the dualities of time and space into our true nature. Our body-n-soul art is simplicity in Nature. We came here to create on the canvas of life. The sacred, living sanctuary we call Earth provides all the tools needed to create the masterpiece that is always a work in progress.

It is critical now that we embody the art of peace and love so that we align with our true selves. We no longer need to play the victim and blame or judge other people and other nations for the ills of the world since we all create it together as one big soul family. We cannot depend on our current educational system to change the state of the economy, government, social, medical, or environmental structures when they all reflect each other. When education teaches how and what to think, instead of *to think* independently, it trains us rather than inspires us. Learning history keeps us from living in the now and creating from the moment. We repeat the past instead of living in the now.

These systems feed conformity, oppression, compliance, and a perceived need for a higher power. When we perceive and believe there is enough for everyone on this Earth, we live in a state of abundance. When we act from that state, everything we need shows up. The experience of our life is who we are in our hearts and minds. We don't find it on television or in so-called expert opinions.

We are powerful miracles of creation, limited only by our beliefs. We are here to take up our staff and walk the road of our own choosing, leading with the heart. To change the world in which we live, we must first unlearn what we've been taught and conditioned to believe and relearn how to think for ourselves. After we come into our individual power, we must live in that power. Become our own innovation, and move it forward. What happens on Earth ripples throughout the Universe for the highest good. And we can all get used to that.

"Abundance is not something we acquire. It is something we create."

~Wayne Dyer, author

Our bodies are ecosystems made up of 100 trillion cells, the majority of which are not of human origin. We host and sustain the same bacteria that live on planet Earth, which sustains and hosts all of us. How we nourish ourselves and how we act affects the whole. Reconnecting to Nature is paramount to discovering true health because it is through this bond that we each embody the innate capacity to heal ourselves. As we accept our true potential as healers our healing vibes ripples out to Earth who heals herself and sends her healing vibes back to us, maintaining balance and sustaining the whole.

Were Nature when we see the Earth as a living being, whose sacred geometry and energy chakra system is reflected in our own being. We coexist in all cultures. We are One in body, mind, and spirit. We come into balance by living in the rhythm of Nature. We come into our power to actively create a new paradigm of reality by using our gifts and living our truth. Truth is simple. The healing journey is all about overcoming duality to become One.

In making the choice of when to begin, there is no time like the present.

Some Personal Heroes

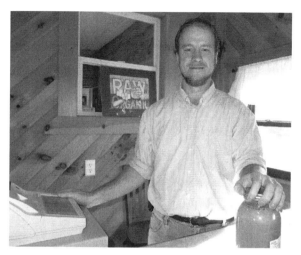

Vernon Hershberger, farmer for the people. Champion for the freedom to choose
real, nutrient-dense foods, November 2012, Wisconsin.

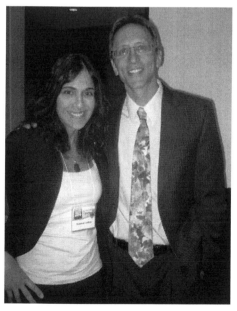

With Dr. Robert Scott Bell, homeopath & the Voice of Health Freedom and Liberty,
Health Freedom Expo, June 2012, Chicago

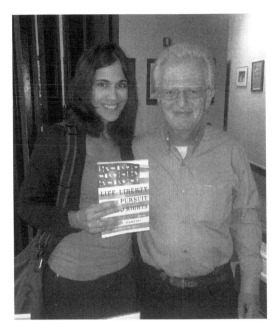

With Author David Gumpert, "Life, Liberty and the Pursuit of Food Right," June 2012, Madison

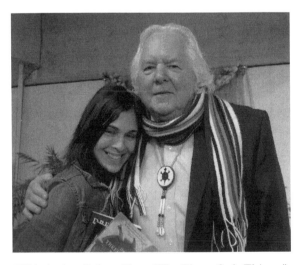

With Author Robert Moss, "The Three Only Things." April 2013, Madison

Heroes Continued...

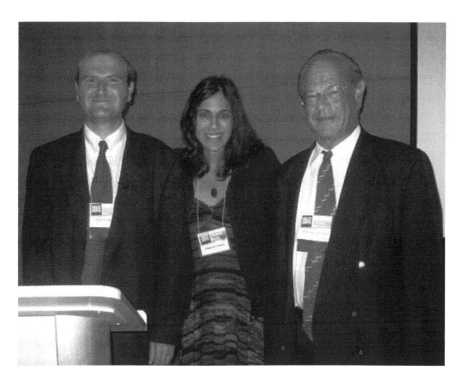

With Mark (right) and son David Geier (left), researchers linking thimerosal in vaccines to rise in autism, Health Freedom Expo, Chicago, June 2012.

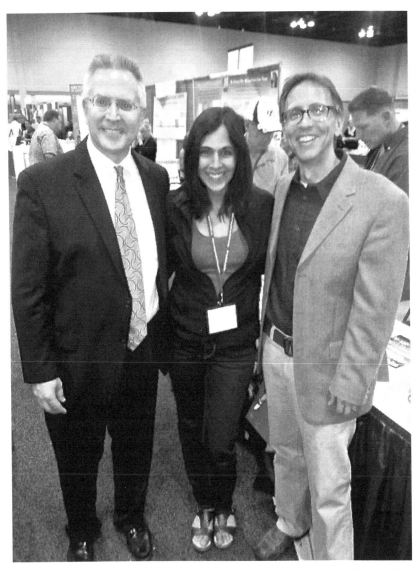

Game Changers: Constitutional Attorney Jonathan Emord (left) Dr. Robert Scott Bell (right); voices of Health Freedom and Liberty, Health Freedom Expo, Chicago, June 2013.

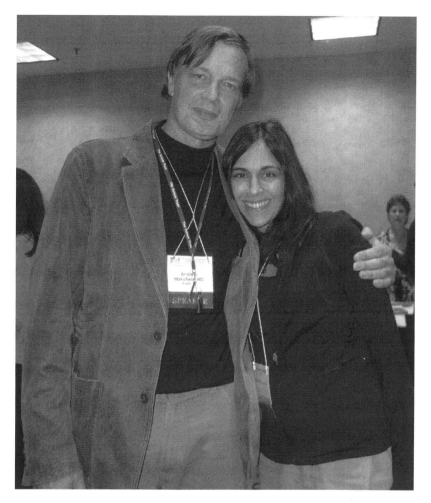

With Dr. Andrew Wakefield (right), gastroenterologist, researcher, humanitarian for truth and healing for children with autism, Wise Traditions Conference, Atlanta, November 2013.

About the Author

Rosanne Lindsay, B.C.N.D., is a writer, mother, and Naturopathic Doctor, certified by the American Naturopathic Medical Certification Board. She is a graduate of Trinity School of Natural Health in Naturopathic Medicine and an advocate for natural health and healing, self-empowerment, and the freedom to choose one's own foods. As a holistic practitioner, she incorporates energy medicine and crystal healing into her practice.

Rosanne believes that if given the tools Nature provides, the body heals itself. This book evolved from her own journey of healing after being diagnosed with "profound hypothyroidism," an acute and severe form of hypothyroidism manifesting in physical symptoms that included mild depression, sluggishness, forgetfulness, cold intolerance, weight gain, constipation, peripheral edema, light sensitivity, and dyspnea (shortness of breath) upon mild exertion, among other symptoms. Using an eclectic mix of dietary changes, nutrition, herbal supplements, minerals, glandulars, energy medicine, acupuncture, yoga, meditation, and a life overhaul, Rosanne discovered that profound healing comes from taking profound measures: digging deep, altering patterns of belief, and working on body, mind, and spirit as one. Through her lifestyle changes, she reversed the condition naturally within less than a year, and discovered her gifts as a healer.

Prior to raising her children, Rosanne earned an M.A. in the field of environmental health science and worked as an Environmental Scientist for the United States Environmental Protection Agency helping to write and enforce air pollution regulations. She has worked in local government and as a volunteer in the Madison, Wisconsin area to protect watersheds against runoff pollution, urban sprawl, the depletion of ground water, and to inform the community about the adverse health impacts which often accompany these changes. She appreciates that our collective health is a direct reflection of the health of our planet. Her passion is to guide and empower others on their own path of health and healing and to teach, that through our connection to Nature, each person has the capacity to heal Self and the planet.

Appendix I

MINERAL FUNCTIONS

Mineral deficiency symptoms and functions of some minerals:[451]

- Calcium – Lack causes bone softening, digestive problems, cramps, aches, pain, fatigue, fear, and indecision. Calcium is one of the most important minerals, required by every cell in the body. Calcium builds and maintains bones, teeth, hormones, and blood; regulates heart rhythm; and buffers acidity, among other things.
- Cobalt – Lack results in pernicious anemia, stunted growth, and nerve damage. Cobalt is a necessary component of red blood cells, many enzymes, and is important to vitamin B12; also necessary for normal growth and appetite.
- Chromium – Lack causes blood sugar imbalance, hardening of arteries, heart disease. Chromium is integral part of many enzymes and hormones, is a co-factor for insulin to move glucose from blood to cells (especially for diabetics), and reduces plaque in those suffering from arteriosclerosis. Chromium GTF deficiency is common in diabetics but may be allergenic to some people unless it is from a whole food source.

- Copper – Lack causes heart abnormalities, osteoporosis, decreased bone marrow density, and low white cell counts, resulting in frequent and severe infections and lowered immune function. Copper is necessary for normal iron metabolism and transport to the bone marrow for red blood cell formation. Copper plays an important role in oxidation-reduction reactions (redox) and in scavenging free radicals. It is important component for many essential enzymes for cell energy production and the formation of strong connective tissue in the heart and blood vessels.
- Iodine – Lack impairs the function of the thyroid gland, resulting in goiter, and thyroid disease (hypothyroidism/hyperthyroidism). Essential for proper growth, energy, and metabolism. Lack of iodine in pregnant mothers can result in cretinism (mental retardation).
- Iron – Lack causes fingernail ridges, flat nails, and exfoliation, slow growing hair, and anemia. Required for hemoglobin; carries oxygen in the blood.
- Magnesium – Lack results in weaknesses of bones, teeth, and muscles and may give rise to heart ailments. Necessary for calcium and vitamin C metabolism and neuromuscular system function.
- Manganese – Lack causes tinnitis in left ear, impotence in men, sexual apathy, lack of muscle strength, allergic reaction to rice. Necessary for enzyme metabolism in carbohydrate, protein, and fat metabolism, improves eyesight, necessary for tissue respiration, bones, and organs.
- Molybdenum – Lack results in sexual impotence in older males and esophageal tumors. Necessary for carbohydrate metabolism.
- Phosphorus – Lack causes arthritis, weakens bones and teeth, causes weight loss. Necessary for calcium metabolism; lecithin and cerebrin synthesis for brain, stimulates hair growth, buffers blood pH, and maintains bone density.
- Potassium – Lack causes weakness of the muscles and paralysis, high blood pressure. It may also cause brittleness of the bones, sterility, and heart ailments. Necessary for blood pH,

fluid balance between cells, muscle tone, nerves, heart action, enzyme reactions; assists kidneys in eliminating blood impurities. It carries electrical chi that nurtures and activates muscles and organ systems.

- Selenium – Lack causes liver damage, muscle degeneration, heart disease, premature aging, and may lead to tumors of digestive tract and other organs. Selenium is a powerful antioxidant, prevents free-radical formation, helps dandruff, protects against mercury toxicity, regenerates liver after damage (cirrhosis), and is essential for the enzyme glutathione peroxidase for glutathione, another powerful antioxidant that is made by every cell to detoxify and clear heavy metals and fight free radicals to reduce inflammation and slow aging.

- Silicon – Lack causes dry brittle hair, skin, and nails. Silicon is essential trace element for connective tissue in bone and cartilage. Silicon-supplemented bones have much higher collagen content than low-silicon bones which promotes faster bone growth as well as more flexible and resilient bodies. Silica is naturally found in the Horsetail herb.

- Sodium – Lack results in bronchial and lung problems. Sodium, is one of three electrolytes, along with potassium and chloride, that is an ion in solution to regulate water in the body and conduct electricity, and is therefore critical to cell function. It is also critical to maintaining calcium in solution, blood and lymph fluidity, eliminating CO_2, and is the main buffer to acidity and against inflammation. Celery, rich in sodium and high in water content and is known to help bring down a fever.

- Sulfur – Lack causes inefficient metabolic processes. Necessary for hair, skin, nails; aids in dissolving acids, improves circulation, normalizes heart action. Present in all cells and necessary in formation of amino acids, synthesis of collagen; increases bile function, has cleansing effect in digestive tract. It is an antidote for fat allergy.[452] Sulfur is also necessary component of the anti-aging antioxidant, glutathione.

- Zinc – Lack causes hair loss, stunted growth, frequent infections, reduced immune function, dry skin, anemia, weight loss. Zinc influences entire hormonal system and glands. Helps tissue function (kidney, liver, pancreas, prostate), protein synthesis, carbohydrate metabolism, and tissue respiration (transports CO from tissues to blood), among other things.

Appendix II

GENERAL PROTOCOLS FOR NATURAL HEALING

1. Heal the Gut and Repopulate with Probiotics
2. Alkalinize & Detoxify

Heal the Gut

An easy and essential protocol to restoring the lining of the small intestine is one designed by homeopath Dr. Robert Scott Bell using colloidal silver and pure aloe vera juice. The first step to boosting the immune system is to heal the gut. Until the holes in the gut are fully healed by restoring the beneficial microbes, no amount of nutrition will be absorbed for energy. Dr. Bell's Silver-Aloe Intestinal healing protocol, which he shares in his lectures and on his radio show, uses silver hydrosol (Sovereign Silver®) because of its remarkable healing properties that are anti-fungal, anti-viral, and anti-bacterial.

Sovereign Silver hydrosol® is an oligodynamic silver made up of positively charged silver ions (cations) that remain unbound to protein and in suspension in a fully active state for assimilation in the body. Its sub-nano particle size and its low silver 10 ppm content mean silver hydrosol is completely safe (vs. other colloidal silver products contaminated with salts at 500+ ppm), and thereby allows for multiple daily doses. The smaller the silver particle size the more potent its energy. Alternatively, ionic silver is an inferior form of neutral silver /silver salt that is dissolved in solution rather than in a colloidal suspension. Higher concentrations of silver are comprised of very high particle size ranges and therefore contain little, if any, charged silver particles. Caution: Using inferior products high in salts and proteins can lead to a condition called Argyria where accumulations can turn the skin blue.

Sovereign Silver® carries up to ten times its atomic weight in oxygen and is safely ingested in small amounts to heal tissues, prevent scar formation, kill viruses and yeast. It can be nebulized for lung infections, sprayed on mucous membranes (nose, eyes), and used as a gel for topical cuts and scrapes.

Silver-Aloe Intestinal Healing Protocol

Adults take ½ oz to 1 oz (15-30 ml) liquid Silver Hydrosol (1/4 oz for children) with same amount of pure aloe vera juice. Drink three times per day prior 45 minutes to meals. Continue for 3 to 4 weeks. For more severe conditions (IBS, Crohn's, chronic digestive disorders) take 4-8 weeks. This form of silver (Sovereign Silver®) is recommended to take away from meals to avoid canceling some of the benefits. Adjunct supplements Dr. Bell recommends include: L-glutamine (amino-acid), silica, and homeopathic Baptisia. Contraindicated with this protocol: Sulfur-based drugs, which bind and prevent absorption of silver.

Repopulate the Gut with Probiotics

Simultaneous to the Silver-Aloe protocol it is important to restore the integrity of immune function at the source (the gut) by adding a non-GMO probiotic once a day before bed. Replenishing good gut flora restores function to digestion, immunity, neurotransmitter production, and endocrine. Once the gut is healed, you can also supplement with a probiotics once a day in the morning away from meals. You can also include probiotic/fermented foods like kimchi, fermented coleslaw/cabbage, kefir, kombucha, etc. Check out the book *Wild Fermentation: The Flavor, Nutrition, and Craft of Live-Culture Foods*, by Sandor Katz.

Alkalinize the Body

The natural world speaks to us through the soil and the plants. All we need to do is listen. Plants grow best in an optimal soil pH of 6.4.

When the soil contains a diverse population of soil microbes, plants do not attract viruses, pests, or disease. The same holds true for humans.

Alkalinizing the body means to push an acidic pH to optimal. This is widely considered to be one of the most important things you can do to. One can self-monitor the body using pH test strips to check acidity of saliva and urine on a daily or weekly basis. Our cells do their best work when the saliva and urine pH measures at 6.4 (range 6.2 – 6.6).[453] According to Dr. Carey Reams's biological theory of ionization, urine pH indicates the efficiency of the gastric juices of the stomach and how efficiently the kidneys are removing toxins from the body and saliva pH indicates the efficiency of liver and pancreatic enzymes. Biological ionization analysis is an excellent metabolic biofeedback tool to show whether one's lifestyle is beneficial or not. It shows that if one's metabolic efficiency is straying from the optimal pH of 6.4, one becomes predisposed to degeneration and disease. On the positive side, it provides specific information (when using a mathematical formula measuring sugar, mineral salts, and cell debris) on the minerals and vitamins not being assimilated into the body's cells so that changes can be made on a holistic level.

Saliva and Urine pH Testing

Anyone can test his own urine and saliva pH. When testing saliva pH, we are looking at the pH of most bodily fluids and conditions before digestion. Saliva pH is a liver strength indicator as saliva conditions come directly from the liver and reflect the potential pH of bile. Saliva pH has twice the effect in value of urine as an energy indicator. The magic number for a morning saliva reading is 6.2 and shouldn't go beyond 6.8. A normal reading during the day is about 6.8.

With saliva readings, you're looking for a change in pH before and after a meal. The saliva of most people registers around 5.5 to 6.0 before meals. If yours is in this range before eating, then goes up after meals, your alkaline reserve is low, meaning your sodium levels are low (sodium is stored in the liver and in muscles), but your body can still meet the demands of eating what you are eating. A saliva pH reading of 6.8 before a meal and 8.0 or higher after a meal is ideal because it equals natural physiological function. A 6.2 before a meal and going higher after a meal, is good. A 5.5 before a meal and going higher after is acceptable with some reserves available. If, however, your saliva reads 5.5 to 5.8 before a meal and there is no change after a meal, then the body is extremely acid, indicating no alkaline reserve.[454]

The urine pH test indicates conditions after digestion. A range of 5.5 to 5.8 pH is the most ideal response if you're eating acid foods (meat, dairy, grains) and indicates a well-stocked alkaline reserve. Alkaline urine following a meal of acid-producing food is a sure sign that the alkaline reserve is depleted. This is ammonia being produced by the body to neutralize the strong acid – not good.[455]

All of the body's fluids (approximately ten gallons) are alkaline by design, except the stomach gastric juices. These include the blood, spinal fluid, saliva, duodenum, feces, urine, liver bile, gall bladder bile, pancreas, the fluids inside and outside cells, and around the joints, organs, and brain. Your cells do constantly produce acid as they function, but this weak acid is removed through the lungs (exhaled) or neutralized as an acid-ash before being removed by the kidneys using the body's alkaline reserve. The main minerals of the alkaline reserve, which act to buffer the acid your cells produce are sodium, potassium, calcium, and magnesium, the main one beings sodium, which is stored primarily in the liver and muscles. The best way to acquire these organic minerals is by eating fruits and vegetables.

Alkalinize with Foods

Eat a diet of eighty percent alkaline foods and twenty percent acid foods for neutral pH balance. An acid body results from emotional stress, toxic overload, nutrient deficiencies, immune reactions or any process that deprives the cells of oxygen and other nutrients. The body will compensate for an acidic pH by using alkaline minerals from alkaline-forming foods from your diet.

The list of alkaline foods includes: fresh, organic raw fruits and vegetables, slightly-cooked vegetables, nuts, seeds, sprouts, juices made from green vegetables, milks from almond, cashew, hemp, and coconut, none of which are processed, pasteurized, irradiated, or genetically modified. Nature-made sweets like maple syrup, brown sugar, raw honey, and cacao also factor into this list. Liquids like apple cider vinegar, green juices, coconut water, water, and probiotic drinks.

Fresh coconut water, straight from the coconut is sterile, has the same electrolyte balance as blood, does not produce heat, does not destroy red blood cells, lowers blood sugar,[456] and is readily accepted by the body. As such, it can be substituted for human plasma (intravenous hydration) in emergencies as was reported with critically ill patients during World War II when saline was low, and in remote regions of the world.[457]

Because even organic foods can lack the necessary minerals for health, herbs, liquid supplements, and homeopathics can assist the body as needed.[458] If enough alkaline foods are not available, the body will raid its own calcium stores from the bones, which can result in osteoporosis, gout from uric acid build-up, and bone spurs, among other conditions. Remember, every cell needs calcium.[459] Imbalance results as the body drains itself of its calcium reserves, doing what is needed to keep itself alive.

Reducing acidic foods like meat, processed dairy, enriched grains, seeds, nuts, as well as caffeine, alcohol, and sugar, while increasing vegetables, greens, and fruits builds the alkaline reserve and ensures you always have enough sodium available. Low-Acid eating means removing all processed junkfood from your diet and your pantry. These empty-calorie foods lower pH (create acidity), deplete minerals, damage the immune system, and create an energy debt in the body, causing the body to use more energy to digest and metabolize these foods than the foods provide in energy:

- No enriched flours (wheat breads, pastas, potatoes, cereal grains)
- No dense protein in the form red meats, pork, poultry
- No processed soy (soy milk, soy protein, soy flour, etc.)
- No processed dairy
- No fried foods, crackers
- No hydrogenated GMO seed oils (canola oil, safflower oil, and sunflower oil)
- No refined sugar (especially high-fructose GMO corn syrup and table sugar)
- No refined salt (use sea salt containing all natural minerals)
- No brominated flour or breads
- No alcohol
- No caffeine
- No fluoridated-chlorinated water

Go Gluten-free

A wheat-free or gluten-free diet is a good place to start when beginning a healing journey. Gluten, like other processed food triggers, all have their initial reactions in the small intestine. For thousands of years, wheat was a nutrient dense food from a living seed. After the industrial revolution and the resulting erosion of soils new technologies took wheat in a new direction in the name of food security.

Between 1944 and 1960. agronomist, Dr. Norman Borlaug served as the Rockefeller Foundation scientist in charge of wheat improvement under the Cooperative Mexican Agricultural Program. Borlaug developed new types of high-yielding, disease resistant wheat plants that sparked the "Green Revolution" in Mexico, Indian and Pakistan.[460] Today more than a quarter of the American diet comes from Borlaug wheat which has continued to change through mechanical, chemical and genetic technologies-to become demineralized and undigestible. Our codependency with this grain – to the exclusion of many others – has resulted in gluten sensitivity for up to ninety percent of the population.[461]

Gluten from wheat, rye, and barley tends to be a central food-link common to all autoimmune disease. Gluten is a glycoprotein made up of gliadin and glutinen. A clue to gluten's action comes from its latin meaning--glue. Modern wheat is difficult to digest due to gluten's disulfide (sulfur-to-sulfur) bonds. Its enhanced properties make it more useful as an industrial adhesive in papier mache, paints, and book binding. In ancient times, wheat was mixed with water to create plaster.

Gluten and Autoimmune Disease

In addition to gliadin and glutinen, wheat gluten has several peptides known to irritate the gut lining. Gluten exorphins are one group with opiate-like properties that act as endocrine disruptors and nervous system antigens. Studies show that a significant percentage of children with autism produce high levels of antibodies to gliadin and cerebellar peptides simultaneously, meaning anti-gliadin antibodies attack brain proteins.[462] The highly respected Cochrane Review did a meta-analysis in 2004 on the evidence of a dairy-wheat-autism connection. Their conclusion and recommendation stated:

"It has been suggested that peptides from gluten and casein may have a role in the origins of autism and that the physiology and psychology of autism might be explained by excessive opioid activity linked to these peptides. Research has reported abnormal levels of peptides in the urine and cerebrospinal fluid of persons with autism. If this is the case, diets free of gluten and /or casein should reduce the symptoms associated with autism."

Parents with autistic kids on a gluten-free, casein-free diet see aggression and self-injury (caused by abdominal pain) cease.

In most people, gluten causes T-cell immune activation in the gut mucosa, which not only reduces the variety of gut bacteria, but also promotes the growth of pro-inflammatory bacteria that can make autoimmune reactions worse over time, causing a cascade of autoimmune conditions.[463] GMO wheat is next on the list to enter the food supply. Based on the evidence on hand, it is worthwhile to implement a wheat and dairy elimination diet when dealing with any autoimmune disease, and if proven beneficial, to substitute them with alternatives.

Detoxing The Organs of Elimination

The main organs of elimination are the liver, colon, lungs, kidneys, skin, and lymph. These natural routes of elimination can lose their ability to function from waste products resulting from cellular metabolism (ammonia, urea, uric acid, carbon dioxide, sulfates, phosphates), as well as from external toxins such as pesticides and chemicals. Symptoms of disease are the result of toxic accumulations in the tissues. Below are some natural methods that can be performed during a cleansing diet or at any time to aid the organs in toxin elimination.

Liver: The enema is the fastest, surest way to detoxify the liver. The enema has become a dirty word in modern life but it is a tool that has been used successfully for thousands of years in many cultures to restore liver function and promote self-healing. As normal stool moves through the colon, it eventually reaches a duct between the sigmoid colon and the liver, at which point toxins are sent to the liver for detoxification. The organic coffee enema is a popular low-volume enema that remains only in the sigmoid colon. The alkaloids in the caffeine stimulate the production of glutathione-S-transferase, the enzyme that helps to drain bile out of the liver to clear liver detox pathways.

Up to three enemas per day can be safely used during healing periods. Water enemas are also used with or without the addition of essential oils, probiotics, or barley greens.

Healing herbs help cleanse the liver. Dandelion is a powerful detoxifier, cleanser, and toner of the entire waste disposal system, that increases secretion and flow of bile into the intestines. Yellow Dock has a laxative action and helps clear congestion in the liver. Yarrow regulates and tones the liver and aids the entire glandular system. Warm lemon water (juice of 1/2 to 1 lemon in 8 to 16 oz. glass of water) before breakfast and bed helps purify and stimulate the liver. Lemon water or limewater liquefies bile while inhibiting excess bile flow. According to A.F. Beddoe, author of "Biological Ionization Principles," the liver produces more enzymes from lemon/lime water than any other food. Chase lemon water with 1 T hydrated liquid bentonite clay in a glass of water. Bentonite Clay is a natural liquid clay supplement that binds toxins in the blood for elimination and should be a part of any healing detox plan.

Other detox tools include: 1) castor oil packs to aid in the detox and elimination of toxins, especially in the liver and gall bladder for a wide range of chronic conditions, 2) two natural amino acids, ornithine and arginine are also used to detox ammonia to alkalinize the body and stimulate liver regeneration (see page 11f. in Hulda Clark's book *The Cure for All Cancers*).

Colon: Colon hydrotherapy, also known as colonics, colon irrigation, or high enema, picks up where enemas leave off by gently flushing all four to five feet of the large intestine with warm water. It is an important tool to assist the body in reversing a wide range of disease conditions. The colon is a hollow muscular organ that moves digestive food and waste by a wavelike motion along the last five feet of the digestive tract, the primary function of which is to absorb water, electrolytes, and some vitamins as well as to prepare and store fecal waste prior to elimination. When both saliva and urine pH are above 6.4, expect constipation, a toxic colon, and a strong likelihood of parasites. A highly toxic colon spills over into the lymph system to cause congestion of the sinuses and upper respiratory system.

Healing herbs like chaparral cleanse the colon, lymphatic system, and liver as well as tone peristaltic muscles to move waste through the colon efficiently. Cascara sagrada is a strong laxative that tones peristaltic muscles and increases the secretion of bile and can be used for short periods. Aloe vera juice is a mild laxative.

Lymph: To move the lymphatic system, jump on a rebounder (38-inch mini trampoline). Unlike the heart, the lymph does not have its own pump as it flows in its own channel next to the blood system. Rebound for three minutes, three times per day. Bouncing oxygenates the blood, tightens the skin, and gives an overall sense of wellness.

Other Hydrotherapy

Detox Baths – Hot baths (slowly increase temperature of water) serve to increase circulation in lower pelvic region where salts accumulate. Warm-hot baths help to eliminate salts and regulate water in the colon. Several detox bath recipes are safe and effective:

- Detox Recipe 1: 1 pound sodium bicarbonate (baking soda) to one pound Epsom salt, to bring body pH to a neutral range by pulling acid out of the body. Use pH strips for urine as guidance after morning and afternoon baths. Urine pH should not go over 8.0 to 8.1.[464]
- Detox Bath Recipe 2: 2 cups Epsom salt, (draws out toxins/ adds magnesium) 1 cup apple cider vinegar (neutralizes pH), ½ cup bentonite clay (stimulates lymphatic's to cleanse skin), and 5-10 drops of a favorite essential oil (lavender, geranium, sandlewood, ylang ylang).
- AeroBath Detox: To oxygenate the entire body quickly using ozonated (O-H) water (available in some spas and healing centers by State).
- Foot Detox Bath: To clear head and lung congestion: 1 T yellow mustard powder in hot water bath that accommodates two feet. Soak for 20 minutes. Can also add cayenne pepper. Soothes sore feet, to boot.
- Radiation Detox Bath: Fill an aluminum pan that is large enough to accommodate both hands opened flat with cold tap water. Stir in ½ cup of baking soda until it is dissolved.
  1. Place both hands in the water opened flat and hold them there for 5 minutes. The palms will become warm as the radiation leaves the body.

2. Leaving the left hand immersed in the water, hold the right hand opened flat outside the water above the left hand and hold for 5 minutes.

3. Switch hands, reversing 3 (above) with the left hand out of the water and the right hand completely immersed in the water.

4. Pour the used water down the drain. Wash the aluminum pan and reserve it for this exercise. 5. Do not use it for anything else. This exercise will remove radiation from your body, alkalinizing it bringing peace and calm to your being.

6. Do this exercise as often as necessary until you no longer feel the effects of the radiation. You will know what the radiation feels like after you have felt the difference from having done the Exercise. (From: Master Dr. Earl W. Blighton in the Holy Order of MANS, 1970a. Shared by Master Valentius).

Detoxing parasites can be accomplished using black walnut as an herbal or extract for one to two weeks or by using the Hulda Clark eighteen-day herbal parasite cleanse with ingredients of black walnut, wormwood, and common cloves. Digestive enzymes like papaya enzyme are also added to aid the liver as it heals.[465]

Skin: Daily dry skin brushing helps remove dead cells from the skin, the second largest organ in surface area of your body (after the lungs). Skin works as a respiratory organ, aids in the elimination of toxic wastes from the body, and will tend to be thinner in an acid situation, which can lead to eczema. Brushing removes dead skin cells, cleanses the pores, stimulates the hormone and oil-producing glands in the skin, and improves circulation to maintain skin function. With healthy skin, one can use far infrared sauna to raise body temperature to sweat out toxins. Vitamin C is a cement chelate that helps hold cells together, which can help reverse sagging skin. If unavailable, the lungs are cannibalized for the benefit of other tissues.

Herbal extracts like Oregon grape, whose berries are rich in Vitamin C, is useful for acne, eczema, and as an ointment is useful for psoriasis. This herb suppresses the growth of yeast and other fungal infections, and has strong anti-inflammatory properties useful in autoimmune disease in tumorous conditions. An essential oil like Tea tree oil is used for all anti-fungal, anti-parasitic conditions externally including warts, ringworm, athlete's foot, chicken pox, insect bites, acne, cuts and scrapes, lice and dandruff, and to soften corns. Tea Tree Oil can be applied directly (1 to 2 drops), mixed with a carrier oil (3 to 5 drops), added to an essential oil diffuser, or added to bathwater (6 drops).[466]

Deep belly breathing helps move stale air out of the lungs, which are important organs of elimination since every time you exhale you breathe out metabolic waste products. When oxygen balance in the body is upset, that interferes with levels of insulin and vitamin C. The best breathing position is on your back. Take some deep, slow inhalations followed by a slow exhalation. Then repeat and forcefully exhale, blow out all remaining air in your lungs. Repeat five cycles.

Lung cleansing herbs include mullein, lungwort, thyme, and elecampane. Essential oils for the lungs include inhaling: pine to open bronchial tubes; rose, sage, and sandlewood for chronic bronchitis, as well eucalyptus, frankincense, marjoram, lavender, spruce, fir, cypress, rosemary, rose, clove, clary sage, hyssop, and helichrysum.[467]

Appendix III

RECOMMENDED READING LIST

Disease Reversal Protocols

"The Gerson Therapy" by Charlotte Gerson and Morton Walker, DPM, Kensington, October 2001

"Outsmart Your Cancer" by Tanya Harter Pierce MA. MFCC, Thoughtworks Publishing, 2nd edition. August 2008.

"A Cancer Battle Plan; Six strategies for beating cancer from recovered hopeless care" by Anne E. Frahm with David J. Frahm, Tarcher, December 1997.

"Cancer Free: Your Guide to Gentle, Non-toxic Healing," by Bill Henderson, Booklocker.com Inc. April 2007.

"How to Fight Cancer and Win" by William L. Fischer, Agora Health Books, October 1992

"Cancer – Step Outside the Box," by Ty Bollinger, Infinity 510 Sqauared Partners, July 2006.

"The Only Answer to Cancer," by Dr. Leonard Coldwell, 21C Publishers, October 2009.

"The Alpha Lipoic Acid Breakthrough" by Burt Berkson, MD, PhD, Harmony, September 1998.

"Phoenix Tears, The Rick Simpson Story" by Rick Simpson, Amazon Digital Services, Inc., September 2013.

"Earthing" by Clinton Ober, Stephen T. Sinatra, MD, Martin Zucker, Basic Health Publications, April 2010.

Food/Diet/Politics

"Putting It All Together: The New Orthomolecular Nutrition" by Abram Hoffer, MD PhD & Morton Walker, DPM with introduction by Linus Pauling, PhD, McGraw-Hill, October 1998.

"The 9 Steps to Keep the Doctor Away" by Dr. Rashid Buttar, GMEC Publishing, June 2010.

"The Earth Diet" by Liana Werner-Gray

"Folk Medicine" by D.D. Jarvis, MD, Fawcett, May 1985

"Nourishing Traditions" by Sally Fallon with Mary G. Enig, PhD, Newtrends Publishing, October, 1999.

"Seeds of Deception" by Jeffrey Smith, Yes! Books; 3rd printing edition, September 1, 2003.

"Dangerous Grains" by James Braly, MD, and Ron Hoggan, MA, Avery Trade, August, 2002.

"Gut and Psychology Syndrome: Natural Treatment for Autism, Dyspraxia, A.D.D. Dyslexia, A.D.H.D., Depression, Schizophrenia" by Natasha Campbell-McBride, Medinform Publishing, November 2010.

"Callous Disregard: Autism and Vaccines –The Truth Behind a Tragedy" by Andrew Wakefield, Skyhorse Publishing, July 2011

"Life, Liberty, and the Pursuit of Food Rights" by David Gumpert

Science and Spirituality

"Biology of Belief" by Bruce H. Lipton PhD, Hay House, November 2007.

"Truth vs. Falsehood" by David R. Hawkins, MD, PhD, Axial Publishing, July 2006.

"Power vs. Force: The Hidden Determinants of Human Behavior" by David R. Hawkins, MD, PhD, Veritas Publishing, May 2012.

"The Holographic Universe" by Michael Talbot, Harper Perennial, September 2011.

"The Field: The Quest for the Secret Force of the Universe" by Lynn McTaggert, Harper perennial, January 2008

"Energy Medicine in Therapeutics and Human Performance" by James Oschman, PhD, Butterworth-Heinemann, July 2003.

"Energy Medicine" by Donna Eden, Jeremy P, Tarcher, August 2008.

"Heal Your Body, A to Z" by Louise Hay, Hay House, 1998.

"The Practical Handbook of Homeopathy" by Colin Griffith, MCH, RS Hom, Watkins, April 2008.

"Hands of Light" by Barbara Ann Brennan, Bantam, May 1988.

Spirituality/Energy/Dreams/Yoga

"The Power of Now: A Guide to Spiritual Enlightenment" by Eckhart Tolle, New World Library, August 2004.

"A New Earth: Awakening to Your Life's Purpose" by Eckhart Tolle, Penguin, January 2008.

"As a Man Thinketh" by James Allen.James Allen Books, September 22, 2013.

"Autobiography of a Yogi" by Paramahansa Yogananda, Self-Realization Fellowship, January, 1998.

"Sacred Signs" by Adrian Calabrese, Ph.D, Liewellyn Publications, February, 2006

"The Three Only Things" by Robert Moss, New World Library, June, 2009

"Yoga for the Body, Mind, and Beyond" by Ravi Singh, White Lion Press, April, 1997.

"Peace with Cancer" by Myron Eschowsky Shoshanna Publications, 2009.

"Shamanic Journeying: A Beginner's Guide" by Sandra Ingerman, Sounds True; June June, 2008

"Wheels of Light" by Rosalyn L. Bruyere, Touchstone Publishing, April, 1994.

Appendix IV

PHYSICIAN'S WARRANTY OF VACCINE SAFETY

I (Physician's name, degree)_____, _____
am a physician licensed to practice medicine in the State/Province
of _____, in the country of _____. My
State/Province license number is _____ , and (if the
USA) my DEA number is _____. My medical specialty is
_____.

I have a thorough understanding of the risks and benefits of all the
medications that I prescribe for or administer to my patients. In
the case of (Patient's name) _____ , age
_____ , whom I have examined, I find that certain risk factors
exist that justify the recommended vaccinations. The following is a
list of said risk factors and the vaccinations that will protect against
them:

Risk Factor _____
Vaccination _____
Risk Factor _____
Vaccination _____
Risk Factor _____
Vaccination _____
Risk Factor _____

Vaccination _____

Risk Factor _____

Vaccination _____

Risk Factor _____

Vaccination _____

I am aware that vaccines typically contain many of the following fillers:
* aluminum hydroxide
* aluminum phosphate
* ammonium sulfate
* amphotericin B
* animal tissues: pig blood, horse blood, rabbit brain,
* dog kidney, monkey kidney,
* chick embryo, chicken egg, duck egg
* calf (bovine) serum
* betapropiolactone
* fetal bovine serum
* formaldehyde
* formalin
* gelatin
* glycerol
* human diploid cells (originating from human aborted fetal tissue)
* hydrolized gelatin
* mercury thimerosol (thimerosal, Merthiolate(r))
* monosodium glutamate (MSG)
* neomycin
* neomycin sulfate
* phenol red indicator
* phenoxyethanol (antifreeze)
* potassium diphosphate
* potassium monophosphate
* polymyxin B
* polysorbate 20
* polysorbate 80
* porcine (pig) pancreatic hydrolysate of casein
* residual MRC5 proteins
* sorbitol
* tri(n)butylphosphate,

* VERO cells, a continuous line of monkey kidney cells, and
* washed sheep red blood

and, hereby, warrant that these ingredients are safe for injection into the body of my patient. I have researched reports to the contrary, such as reports that mercury thimerosal causes severe neurological and immunological damage, and find that they are not credible.

I am aware that some vaccines have been found to have been contaminated with Simian Virus 40 (SV 40) and that SV 40 is causally linked by some researchers to non-Hodgkin's lymphoma and mesotheliomas in humans as well as in experimental animals. I hereby warrant that the vaccines I employ in my practice do not contain SV40 or any other live viruses. (Alternately, I hereby warrant that said SV40 virus or other viruses pose no substantive risk to my patient.)

I hereby warrant that the vaccines I am recommending for the care of (Patient's name) _____ _____
do not contain any tissue from aborted human babies (also known as "fetuses").

In order to protect my patient's well being, I have taken the following steps to guarantee that the vaccines I will use will contain no damaging contaminants.

STEPS TAKEN: _____
_____
_____
_____
_____

I have personally investigated the reports made to the VAERS (Vaccine Adverse Event Reporting System) and state that it is my professional opinion that the vaccines I am recommending are safe for administration to a child under the age of 5 years.

The bases for my opinion are itemized on Exhibit A, attached hereto, -- "Physician's Bases for Professional Opinion of Vaccine Safety." (Please itemize each recommended vaccine separately along with the bases for arriving at the conclusion that the vaccine is safe for administration to a child under the age of 5 years.)

The professional journal articles I have relied upon in the issuance of this Physician's Warranty of Vaccine Safety are itemized on Exhibit B, attached hereto, -- "Scientific Articles in Support of Physician's Warranty of Vaccine Safety."

The professional journal articles that I have read which contain opinions adverse to my opinion are itemized on Exhibit C, attached hereto, -- "Scientific Articles Contrary to Physician's Opinion of Vaccine Safety"

The reasons for my determining that the articles in Exhibit C were invalid are delineated in Attachment D, attached hereto, -- "Physician's Reasons for Determining the Invalidity of Adverse Scientific Opinions."

Hepatitis B

I understand that 60 percent of patients who are vaccinated for Hepatitis B will lose detectable antibodies to Hepatitis B within 12 years. I understand that in 1996 only 54 cases of Hepatitis B were reported to the CDC in the 0-1 year age group. I understand that in the VAERS, there were 1,080 total reports of adverse reactions from Hepatitis B vaccine in 1996 in the 0-1 year age group, with 47 deaths reported.

I understand that 50 percent of patients who contract Hepatitis B develop no symptoms after exposure. I understand that 30 percent will develop only flu-like symptoms and will have lifetime immunity. I understand that 20 percent will develop the symptoms of the disease, but that 95 percent will fully recover and have lifetime immunity.

I understand that 5 percent of the patients who are exposed to Hepatitis B will become chronic carriers of the disease. I understand that 75 percent of the chronic carriers will live with an asymptomatic infection and that only 25 percent of the chronic carriers will develop chronic liver disease or liver cancer, 10-30 years after the acute infection. The following scientific studies have been performed to demonstrate the safety of the Hepatitis B vaccine in children under the age of 5 years.

_____
_____
_____
_____

_____
_____
_____
_____

In addition to the recommended vaccinations as protections against the above cited risk factors, I have recommended other non-vaccine measures to protect the health of my patient and have enumerated said non-vaccine measures on Exhibit D, attached hereto, "Non-vaccine Measures to Protect Against Risk Factors" I am issuing this Physician's Warranty of Vaccine Safety in my professional capacity as the attending physician to (Patient's name) _____.

Regardless of the legal entity under which I normally practice medicine, I am issuing this statement in both my business and individual capacities and hereby waive any statutory, Common Law, Constitutional, UCC, international treaty, and any other legal immunities from liability lawsuits in the instant case. I issue this document of my own free will after consultation with competent legal counsel whose name is _____, an attorney admitted to the Bar in the State/Province of _____.

_____ (Name of Attending Physician)

_____ L.S. (Signature of Attending Physician)

Signed on this _____ day of _____ A.D. _____

Witness: _____ Date: _____

Notary Public: _____ Date: _____

References

1   Orgel, L. E., and F. H. C. Crick. "Selfish DNA: The Ultimate Parasite." *Nature* 284, no. 5757 (1980): 604-07. doi:10.1038/284604a0.

2   Thomas, Chris. *Synthesis.* Llandysul: Fortynine Publishers, 2011.

3   Jonathan Wells, *The Myth of Junk DNA.* Seattle, WA: Discovery Institute, 2011.

4   Thomas, Chris, Synthesis, p.14.

5   Katz, Michael. *Wisdom of the Gemstone Guardians.* Portland, Or.: Natural Healing Press, 2005.

6   Eshowskey, Myron. *Shamanic Practice Supervision Group.* November 23, 2013. Workshop I, Wisconsin, Madison.

7   Kirsch, Irving, and Guy Sapirstein. "Listening to Prozac but Hearing Placebo: A Meta-analysis of Antidepressant Medication." *Prevention & Treatment* 1, no. 1 (July 1998). doi:10.1037//1522-3736.1.1.12a.

8   Wechsler, M.E., J.M. Kelley, I.O.E. Boyd, S. Dutile, et al. "Active or Placebo Albuterol, Sham Acupuncture or No Treatment in Asthma." *New England Journal of Medicine* 365 (2001): 119-26.

9   Mondaini, Nicola, Paolo Gontero, Gianluca Giubilei, Giuseppe Lombardi, et al. "Finasteride 5 mg and Sexual Side Effects: How Many of These Are Related to a Nocebo Phenomenon?" *The Journal of Sexual Medicine* 4, no. 6 (November 2007): 1708-712. doi:10.1111/j.1743-6109.2007.00563.x.

10 Strauss, D. C., and J. M. Thomas. "What Does the Medical Profession Mean By "Standard of Care?"" *Journal of Clinical Oncology* 27, no. 32 (November 06, 2009): E192-193. doi:10.1200/JCO.2009.24.6678.

11 Gary Null, *Death by Medicine.* Mount Jackson, VA: Praktikos, 2010.

12 12 Prasad, Vinay, Andrae Vandross, Caitlin Toomy, Michael Cheung et al. "A Decade of Reversal: An Analysis of 146

Contraindicated Medical Practices." *Mayo Clinic Proceedings* 88. no. 8 (2013): 790-98.

13   Ji, Sayer. "Millions Wrongly Treated for 'Cancer,' National Cancer Institute Panel Confirms - Page 2." Millions Wrongly Treated for 'Cancer,' National Cancer Institute. July 31, 2013. Accessed October 23, 2013. http://www.greenmedinfo.com/blog/millions-wrongly-treated-cancer-national-cancer-institute-panel-confirms?page=2.

14   *The Precautionary Principle: A Common Sense Way to Protect Public Health and the Environment.* Report. Assessed January 2000. Science and Environmental Health Network.

15   Jeremy Laurance. "Drug Giants Fined $11bn for Criminal Wrongdoing." The Independent. September 20, 2013. Accessed October 15, 2013. http://www.independent.co.uk/life-style/health-and-families/health-news/drug-giants-fined-11bn-for-criminal-wrongdoing-8157483.html.

16   Kevin Outterson, J.D., LL.M. "Punishing Health Care Fraud ~ Is the GSK Settlement Sufficient?" *N Engl J Med*, 367 (September 20, 2012): 1082-1085. DOI: 10.1056/NEJMp1209249.

17   Jonathan W. Emord, *Global Censorship of Health Information.* Washington, D.C.: Sentinel Press, 2010.

18   Turnbaugh PJ, Ley RE, Hamady M, Fraser-Liggett CM, Knight R, and Gordon JI. "The Human Microbiome Project." *Nature.* 2007 449, no. 7164 (October 18, 2007): 804-810. 804-10. doi:10.1038/nature06244.

19   Mullard, A. "Microbiology: The inside Story." *Nature* 453 (2008): 575-80.

20   Herper, M. "Germs That Are Good For You." *Forbes.* 1 January 1, 2010. www.forbes.com/2010/01/11/bacteria-obesity-diabetes-lifestyle-health-healthy-germs.html.

21   Schloss, Patrick David, and Jo Handelsman. "Toward a Census of Bacteria in Soil." *PLoS Computational Biology* Preprint. 2006 (2005): E92.

22   Jensen, Marni N. "Good Dirt: Finding New Antibiotics in Farm Soil,"| *Vaccination News.* May 21, 2003. Accessed September 28, 2013. http://www.vaccinationnews.com/dailynews/2003/June/06/GoodDirtFindingNew6.htm.

23 Harrington, Carl R. "A Short-oligonucleotidemicroarray That Allows Improved Detection of Gastrointestinal Tract Microbial Communities." *BMC Microbiology,* 8, no. 195 (2008).

24 Samuel, BS, Shaito A, Motoike T, Rey FE, Backhed F. et al. "Effects of the Gut Microbiome on Host Adiposity Are Modulated by the Short-chain Fatty-acid Binding G Protein-coupled Receptor, Gpr41." *Proceedings of the National Academy of Sciences* 105, no. 43 (2008): 16767-6772.

25 Barr, J.J. Auro, R. Furlan, M. Whiteson, K.L. Erb, M.L. Pogliano, J. et al. "Bacteriophage adhering to mucus provide a non–host-derived immunity," PNAS. *Microbiology.* May 20, 2013. doi:10.1073/pnas.1305923110

26 Elizabeth Lipski. *Leaky Gut Syndrome: What to Do about a Health Threat That Can Cause Arthrities, Allergies and a Host of Other Illnesses.* New Canaan, CT: Keats Pub., 1998.

27 Morones-Ramirez, J. R., Winkler, J.A. Spina, C.S., and Collins, J.J. "Silver Enhances Antibiotic Activity Against Gram-Negative Bacteria." *Sci. Transl.* 5, no.190ra81 (2013).

28 Turnbaugh, P., F. Backhed, L. Fulton, and J. Gordon. "Diet-Induced Obesity Is Linked to Marked but Reversible Alterations in the Mouse Distal Gut Microbiome." *Cell Host & Microbe* 3, no.4 (August 17, 2008): 213-23. Doi:10.1016/j.chom.2008.02.015.

29 Tsai, Franklin, and Walter J. Coyle. "The Microbiome and Obesity: Is Obesity Linked to Our Gut Flora?" *Current Gastroenterology Reports* 11, no. 4 (August 11, 2009): 307-13. doi:10.1007/s11894-009-0045-z.

30 Collins, Stephen M., Zane Kassam, and Premysl Bercik. "The Adoptive Transfer of Behavioral Phenotype via the Intestinal Microbiota: Experimental Evidence and Clinical Implications." *Current Opinion in Microbiology* 16, no. 3 (2013): 240-45.

31 Stein, Rob. "Gut Bacteria Might Guide The Workings Of Our Minds." NPR. November 18, 2013. Accessed November 20, 2013. http://www.npr.org/blogs/health/2013/11/18/244526773/gut-bacteria-might-guide-the-workings-of-our-minds?utm_content=socialflow.

32 Cani, P. D., J. Amar, M.A. Iglesias, and M. Poggi. "Metabolic Endotoxemia Initiates Obesity and Insulin Resistance." *Diabetes* 56, no.7 (2007): 1761-772.

33 Watve, M. Parab, S. Jogdand, P. and Keni, S. "Aging may be a conditional strategic choice and not an inevitable outcome for bacteria." 103, no. 40 (2006): 14831-14835. *Cell Biology.* published ahead of print September 25, 2006, doi:10.1073/pnas.0606499103

34 Watve MG , Shejwal V , Sonawane C , Rahalkar M , Matapurkar A , Shouche Y , Patole M , Phadnis N , Champhenkar A , Damle K , et al. "The 'K' selected oligophilic bacteria: a key to uncultured diversity?" *Curr Sci* 78, no. 12 (2000) :1535–1542.

35 Ley, R. E. "Obesity Alters Gut Microbial Ecology." *Proceedings of the National Academy of Sciences* 102.31 (2005): 11070-1075.

36 Kalliomaki, M., MC Collado, S. Salminen et al. "Early Differences in Fecal Microbiota Composition in Children May Predict Overweight." *Am J Clin Nutr* 87, no. 3 (2008): 534-38.

37 Roper, F., and M.J. Blazer. "The Effect of H. Pylori Eradication on Meal-associated Changes in Plasma Ghrelin and Leptin." *BMC Gastroenterol* 11, no. 37 (2011).

38 Berkey, C. S. "Milk, Dairy Fat, Dietary Calcium, and Weight Gain: A Longitudinal Study of Adolescents." *Archives of Pediatrics and Adolescent Medicine* 159, no.6 (2005): 543-50.

39 Afrc, R. Fuller. "Probiotics in Man and Animals." *Journal of Applied Microbiology* 66, no. 5 (1989): 365-78.

40 Lee, et al. "Human Originated Bacteria, Lactobacillus Rhamonosus PL60, Produce Conjugated Linoleic Acid and Show Anti-obesity Effects in Diet-induced Obese Mice." *Biochem Biophys Acta.* 1761, no. 7 (2006): 736-44.

41 Karlsson, Caroline L. J., Göran Molin, Frida Fåk, and Marie-Louise Johansson Hagslätt. "Effects on Weight Gain and Gut Microbiota in Rats given Bacterial Supplements and a High-energy-dense Diet from Fetal Life through to 6 Months of Age." *British Journal of Nutrition* 106, no. 06 (2011): 887-95.

42 Raoult, D. "Obesity Pandemics and the Modification of Digestive Bacterial Flora." *European Journal of Clinical Microbiology & Infectious Diseases* 27, no .8 (April 2008): 631-34.

43 Mary Ruebush, *Why Dirt Is Good: 5 Ways to Make Germs Your Friends.* New York: Kaplan Pub., 2009.

44 Romagnani, Sergio. "Immunologic Influences on Allergy and the TH1/TH2 Balance." *Journal of Allergy and Clinical Immunology* 113, no .3 (2004): 395-400.

45 Hersoug, L. "A Reformulation of the Hygiene Hypothesis: Maternal Infectious Diseases Confer Protection against Asthma in the Infant." *Medical Hypotheses* 67, no. 4 (2006): 717-20.

46 Debarry, J., MSc, G. Holger, PhD, A. Hanuszkiewicz, MSc, N. Dickgreber, MSc, et al. "Acinetobacter Lwoffii and Lactococcus Lactis Strains Isolated from Farm Cowsheds Possess Strong Allergy-protective Propertie." *Journal of Allergy & Clinical Immunology* 119, no. 6 (2007): 1514-521.

47 Von Mutius, Erika, and Donata Vercelli. "Farm Living: Effects on Childhood Asthma and Allergy." *Nature Reviews Immunology.* 10 (2010): 861-868.

48 Waser, M., K. B. Michels, C. Bieli, H. Flöistrup, et al. "Inverse Association of Farm Milk Consumption with Asthma and Allergy in Rural and Suburban Populations across Europe." *Clinical & Experimental Allergy* 37, no .5 (2007): 661-70.

49 MacNeill, S.J., B. Sozanska, A. Debinska, and A. Kosmeda. "Asthma and Allergies: Is the Farming Environment (still) Protective in Poland? The GABRIEL Advanced Studies." *Allergy* 68, no. 6 (June 2013): 771-91.

50 Cowan, Thomas S., Sally Fallon, and Jaimen McMillan. *The Fourfold Path to Healing: Working with the Laws of Nutrition, Therapeutics, Movement and Meditation in the Art of Medicine.* Washington D.C.: NewTrends Pub., 2004.

51 Lipski R. *Leaky Gut Syndrome.*

52 Wendel, Paul. *Standardized Naturopathy: The Science and Art of Natural Healing.* Brooklyn, NY: Wendel, 1951.

53 Robert J. Thiel *Naturopathy for the 21st Century: Combining Old and New.* Warsaw, IN: W Whitman Publications, 2001.

54 Thiel, R. *Naturopathy.*

55 Ullman, Dana. *Discovering Homeopathy: Medicine for the 21st Century.* Berkeley, CA: North Atlantic, 1988.

56 Bernard Jensen, PhD., *Iridology, the Science and Practice in the Healing Arts.* 2nd Edition. Whitman Publications. Indiana. 2007.

57 Carey A. Reams. *Choose! Life or Death: The Reams Biological Theory of Ionization.* Harrison, AR: New Leaf, 1978.

58 Alexander Beddoe, *Biologic Ionization as applied to human nutrition*, 6ᵗʰ ed. Wendell W. Whitman Company. Warsaw. 2002.

59 NS Davis. In: History of the American Medical Association from its organization up to January 1855. Butler SW, editor. Philadelphia: Lippincott, Grambo and Co; 1855.

60 Beck, A. H. "The Flexner Report and the Standardization of American Medical Education." *JAMA* 291, no. 17 (2004): 2139-140. doi:10.1001/jama.291.17.2139.

61 Duffy, Thomas P., MD. "The Flexner Report - 100 Years Later." *Yale J Biol Med.* 84, no. 3 (2011): 269-76.

62 Hiatt, Mark D.; Christopher Stockton. "The Impact of the Flexner Report on the Fate of Medical Schools in North America After 1909." *Journal of American Physicians and Surgeons* (2003) 8, no. 2. Retrieved 24 November 2012.

63 Johnson, Claire, DC, and Bart Green, DC. "100 Years After the Flexner Report." *J Chiropr Educ.* 24.2 (2010): 145-52.

64 Cook, Trevor. *Samuel Hahnemann: The Founder of Homeopathic Medicine*. England: Thorsons, 1981. P 144.

65 Jugal Kishore, "Homeopathy: The Indian Experience." World Health Forum. 3(1983): 107.

66 Nguyen, Long T., Roger B. Davis, Ted J. Kaptchuk, and Russell S. Phillips. "Use of Complementary and Alternative Medicine and Self-Rated Health Status: Results from a National Survey." *Journal of General Internal Medicine* 26.4 (2011): 399-404.

67 Nahin, RL, Barnes PM, Stussman BJ, and Bloom B. Costs of Complementary and Alternative Medicine (CAM) and Frequency of Visits to CAM Practitioners: United States, 2007 [360KB PDF]. National health statistics reports; no 18. Hyattsville, MD: National Center for Health Statistics. 2009.

68 IOM. "Adverse Events Associated with Childhood Vaccines: Evidence Bearing on Causality. Washington, D.C." *National Academy Press*, 1994a.

69 Sela M, Arnon R. "Synthetic approaches to vaccines for infectious and autoimmune diseases." *Vaccine* (1992):10:991–999.

70 Westall FC, Root-Bernstein RS. "An explanation of prevention and suppression of experimental allergic encephalomyelitis." *Molecular Immunology* (1983): 20:169–177.

71 Berkower, Ira, Hira Nakhasi, Henry McFarland, and Burton Waisbren. *Vaccine Safety Forum: Summaries of Two Workshops (1997) Institute of Medicine (IOM).* National Academies Press, 1997.

72 Miller JFAP, Morahan G, Allison J. "Extrathymic acquisitions of tolerance by T lymphocytes. Cold Spring Harbor" Symposium on Quantitative Biology 1989: LIV:807–813.

73 MacArthur, A. C., M. L. McBride, J. J. Spinelli, and S. Tamaro, et al. "Risk of Childhood Leukemia Associated with Vaccination, Infection, and Medication Use in Childhood: The Cross-Canada Childhood Leukemia Study." *American Journal of Epidemiology* 167, no. 5 (December 12, 2007): 598-606. doi:10.1093/aje/kwm339.

74 Randall Neustaedter and Randall Neustaedter. *The Vaccine Guide: Making an Informed Choice.* Berkeley, CA: North Atlantic, 1996.

75 Belongia, E. A., and A. L. Naleway. "Smallpox Vaccine: The Good, the Bad, and the Ugly." *Clinical Medicine & Research* 1, no. 2 (April 01, 2003): 87-92. doi:10.3121/cmr.1.2.87.

76 Anderson, Gordon W., and Audrey E. Skaar. "Poliomyelitis Occurring after Antigen Injections." *Pediatric* 7.6 (1951): 741-59.

77 Peterson, L.J. M.S.P.H.; Benson, W.W. M.P.H.; Graeber, F.O. "Vaccine-Induce Poliomyelitis in Idaho, Preliminary report of Experience with Salk Poliomyelitis vaccine." M.D. *JAMA.* 1955:159 no. 4 (1955): 241-244.

78 Bayly, Maurice Beddow. *The Story of the Salk Anti-poliomyelitis Vaccine.* London: National Anti-Vivisection Society, 1956.

79 Samuel, R. "Persisting Poliomyelitis after High Coverage with Oral Poliovaccine." *The Lancet* 341, no. 8849 (April 1993): 903. doi:10.1016/0140-6736(93)93117-J.

80 McBean, Eleanor. *The Hidden Dangers in Polio Vaccine.* Mokelumne Hill, CA: Health Research, 1956.

81 Nathanson, N. The Wyeth Report: An Epidemiological Investigation of the Occurrence of Poliomyelitis in Association with Certain Lots of Wyeth Vaccine. August 31, 1955.

82 Nathanson, N. The Wyeth Report: An Epidemiological Investigation of the Occurrence of Poliomyelitis in Association with Certain Lots of Wyeth Vaccine. March 1957.

83 Strebel, P,M., R.W. Sutter, S.L. Cochl, E.W. Brink, et al. "Epidemiology of Poliomyelitis in the United States One Decade after the Last Reported Case of Indigenous Wild Virus-associated Disease." *Clinical Infectious Diseases* 2 (1992): 568-79.

84 "Polio Vaccine: What You Need to Know." *Polio Vaccine and Immunization Information.* CDC, n.d. Web. 21 July 2009.

85 Neil Z. Miller. *Immunization Theory vs. Reality: Exposé on Vaccinations.* Santa Fe, NM: New Atlantean Press, 1996.

86 *Vaccination: The Hidden Truth.* Directed by Viera Scheibner, Ph.D. Performed by Drs. Isaac Golden, David Ritchie, Archie Kalokerinos, Matt Donohoe. Turramurra et al. Australia: Vaccination Information Service, 1998. DVD.

87 Vashisht, Neetu, and Jacob Puliyel. "Polio Programme: Let Us Declare Victory and Move on." *Indian Journal of Medical Ethics* 9, no. 2 (April/May 2012): 114-17.

88 Humphries, Suzanne, MD. CDC and Friends Sprinting Towards the Polio "Finish Line," by Suzanne Humphries, MD. *International Medical Council on Vaccination.* Web. 09 Sept. 2013.

89 Ghosh, Abantika. "Acute Flaccid Paralysis Cases on the Rise in UP, Bihar." The Indian Express. June 18, 2012. Accessed November 03, 2013. http://www.indianexpress.com/news/acute-flaccid-paralysis-cases-on-the-rise-in-up-bihar/963294/1.

90 Gabliks J., Studies of Biologically Active Agents in Cells and Tissue Cultures: Part 1. Annual Progress Report, U.S. Army Medical Research and Development Command. 1966, p. 10.

91 Aufderheide, J., WWII Military Handbook Reveals Pesticide Chemicals Used In Infant Vaccines. VacTruth.com. Sept. 10, 2011.

92 Aufderheide, J., Vaccine Ingredients: Non-ionic Surfactants (Tween 80, Triton X-100, Nonoxynol -9). VacTruth.com. Aug. 23, 2011.

93 Poliomyelitis. Papers and Discussions Presented at the First International Poliomyelitis Conference. Third Session – Tuesday July 13, 1948. J.B. Lippincott Co., Chicago. p. 119.

94 Aycock, W.L. and Luther, E.H., "The occurrence of poliomyelitis following tonsillectomy." *New Engl. J. Med.,* 200 (1929): 164.

95 Aycock, W.L. "Tonsillectomy in Poliomyelitis." *JAMA.* 125, no 14 (1944): 990. doi: 10.1001/jama.1944.02850320048022

96 Eggermont, A. M.M. "Immunostimulation Versus Immunosuppression after Multiple Vaccinations: The Woes of Therapeutic Vaccine Development." *Clinical Cancer Research* 15, no. 22 (2009): 6745-747.

97 Klenner, F. "Massive doses of Vitamin C and the virus disease." *Southern Medicine and Surgery* 103, no. 4 (1951): 101-7.

98 Sandler, Benjamin Pincus. *Diet Prevents Polio.* [Milwaukee]: Lee Foundation for Nutritional Research, 1951.

99 Nakken, Sheri, MA. "Polio Vaccine Page 2." Vaccine/Vaccination/Immunization Dangers. June 15, 2000. Accessed October 22, 2013. http://www.nccn.net/~wwithin/polio2.htm.

100 Glen Dettman, Archie Kalokerinos, and Ian Dettman. *Vitamin C: Nature's Miraculous Healing Missile.* Melbourne, Australie: F. Todd, 1993.

101 "Taking the Breath Out of Asthma (Understanding Asthma – Part II)." *DrGangemicom.* Web. 09 Sept. 2013.

102 Confidential To Regulatory Authorities – Biological Clinical Safety and Pharmacovgilance – GlaxoSmithKline Research and Development Avenue Fleming 20 1300 Wavre Belgium http://ddata.over-blog.com/xxxyyy/3/27/09/71/2012-2013/confid.pdf - See more at: http://vactruth.com/2012/12/16/36-infants-dead-after-vaccine/#sthash.PTsqE6oP.dpuf

103 Kessler, David A., M.D., N.D. "Introducing MEDWatch A New Approach to Reporting Medication and Device Adverse Effects and Product Problems." *JAMA: The Journal of the American Medical Association* 269, no. 21 (1993): 2765-768.

104 Miller, Neil Z. *Immunization Theory vs. Reality: Exposé on Vaccinations.* Santa Fe, NM: New Atlantean Press, 1996.

105 Carbone M, Pass H.I., Rizzo P et al. "Simian virus 40-like DNA sequences in human pleural mesothelioma." *Oncogene 9 (*1994): 1781-1790.

106 Elmishad AG, Bocchetta M, Pass HI, Carbone M. Polio vaccines, SV40 and human tumours, an update on false positive and false negative results. *Dev Biol* (Basel) 123 (2006): 109–132.

107 Vilchez, R., C. Madden, C. Kozinetz, S. Halvorson, et al. "Association between Simian Virus 40 and Non-Hodgkin Lymphoma." *The Lancet* 359, no. 9309 (March 09, 2002): 817-23. doi:10.1016/S0140-6736(02)07950-3.

108 NIH. Infectious Diseases. "NIH Tests Novel Vaccine Made from Weakened Malaria Parasites." News release, January 19, 2012. US Department of Health and Human Services. Accessed October 10, 2013. http://www.niaid.nih.gov/news/newsreleases/2012/Pages/MalariaVRC312.aspx.

109 "UK Firm Seeks to Market World's First Malaria Vaccine." *BBC News*. October 8, 2013. Accessed October 10, 2013. http://www.bbc.co.uk/news/health-24431510.

110 Margaret J. Mackinnon, Andrew F. Read. "Immunity Promotes Virulence Evolution in a Malaria Model." *PLoS Biology*. 2 no. 9 (2004): e230 DOI: 10.1371/journal.pbio.0020230

111 Stevenson, Heidi. "Swine Flu Vaccine Caused Narcolepsy in Thousands: BMJ Claim." Gaia Health. March 6, 2013. Accessed October 10, 2013. http://gaia-health.com/gaia-blog/2013-03-06/swine-flu-vaccine-caused-narcolepsy-in-thousands-bmj-claim/.

112 Collignon, P., P. Doshi, and T. Jefferson. "Ramifications of Adverse Events in Children in Australia." *Bmj* 340, no. Jun09 3 (June 09, 2010): C2994. doi:10.1136/bmj.c2994.

113 Moro, Pedro, Naomi Tepper, Lisa A. Grohskopf, and Claudia Vellozi. "Safety of Seasonal Influenza and Influenza A (H1N1) 2009 Monovalent Vaccines in Pregnancy." *Expert Reviews of Vaccines* 8, no. 8 (August 2012): 911-21. doi:DOI 10.1586/erv.12.72.

114 Christian, L. M. Iams, J.D. Porter, K. Glaser, R. "Inflammatory responses to trivalent influenza virus vaccine among pregnant women." *Vaccine*. September, 2011.

115 Benjamin J. Cowling, Vicky J. Fang, Hiroshi Nishiura, Kwok-Hung Chan, Sophia Ng, Dennis K. M. Ip, Susan S. Chiu, Gabriel M. Leung, and J. S. Malik Peiris "Increased risk of non-influenza respiratory virus infections associated with receipt of inactivated influenza vaccine." *Clin Infect Dis*. (March 15, 2012) doi:10.1093/cid/cis307

116 Kiniry, Erika, MPH et al. *Interim Adjusted Estimates of Seasonal Influenza Vaccine Effectiveness ~ United States, February 2013*. Report no. 62(07). February 22, 2013. Accessed October 20, 2013. http://www.cdc.gov/mmwr/preview/mmwrhtml/mm6207a2.htm.

117 Cervera R, Piette JC, Font J, et al. "Antiphospholipid syndrome: Clinical and immunologic manifestations and patterns of disease

expression in a cohort of 1,000 patients." *Arthritis Rheum* 46 (2002): 1019–1027.

118 Shoenfeld Y. "Systemic antiphospholipid syndrome." *Lupus* 12 (2003): 497–498.

119 Doshi, Peter, PhD. "Influenza: Marketing Vaccines by Marketing Disease." *BMJ* 346 (2013): F3037.

120 Jefferson, T., C. Di Pietrantonj, A. Rivetti, and G.A. Bawazeer. "Vaccines for Preventing Influenza in Healthy Adults." *Cochrane Database Syst Rev* 7 (July 7, 2010): CD001269. doi:10.1002/14651858. CD001269.pub4.

121 Leib, Lee H., M.D. "Letter to Hospital Authorities on Mandatory Influenza Vaccination." *Journal of American Physicians and Surgeons Journal of American Physicians and Surgeons* 18, no. 2 (2013).

122 Marin, M., P. Quinlisk, T. Shimabukuro, and C. Sawhney. "Mumps Vaccination Coverage and Vaccine Effectiveness in a Large Outbreak among College Students ~ Iowa, 2006." Vaccine 26, no. 29-30 (July 04, 2008): 3601-607. doi:10.1016/j.vaccine.2008.04.075.

123 Dayan, Gustavo H., and Steven Rubin. "Mumps Outbreaks in Vaccinated Populations: Are Available Mumps Vaccines Effective Enough to Prevent Outbreaks?" *Clinical Infectious Diseases* 47, no. 11 (2008): 1458-467. doi:10.1086/591196.

124 De Serres, G., N. Boulianne, F. Meyer, and B. J. Ward. "Measles Vaccine Efficacy during an Outbreak in a Highly Vaccinated Population: Incremental Increase in Protection with Age at Vaccination up to 18 Months." Epidemiology and Infection 115, no. 02 (1995): 315. doi:10.1017/S0950268800058441.

125 Chen, R. et al., "An Explosive point-source measles outbreak in a highly vaccinated population modes of transmission and risk factors for disease." *Am. J. Epidemiol.* 129, no. 1 (1989): 173-182.

126 De Melker HE, Conyn-van Spaendonck MA, Rumke HC, van Wijngaarden JK, Mooi FR, and Schellekens JF. "Pertussis in The Netherlands: an outbreak despite high levels of immunization with whole-cell vaccine." *Emerg Infect Dis* 3, no. 2 (1997): 175-178.

127 Grilc E, Pirnat N. "Pertussis outbreak in recently vaccinated children in a kindergarten in Ljubljana during a resurgence in pertussis incidence." *Eurosurveillance.* 10, no. 33. (August 18, 2005).

128 Mooi F R, van LooIHM, King A. "Adaptation of Bordetella pertussis to Vaccination: A Cause for its Reemergence?" *Emerging Infectious Diseases.* 7, no. 3 (June 2001).

129 Johnston, Lucy. "Revealed, Most Compelling Evidence Yet of MMR Danger." Sunday Express (UK), October 6, 2002.

130 Kramer, Reuben. "Wednesday, June 27, 2012Last Update: 10:32 AM PT." Courthouse News Service. June 27, 2012. Accessed November 16, 2013. http://www.courthousenews.com/2012/06/27/47851.htm.

131 Adams, Mike. "Merck Vaccine Fraud Exposed by Two Merck Virologists; Company Faked Mumps Vaccine Efficacy Results for over a Decade, Says Lawsuit." NaturalNews. June 28, 2012. Accessed November 16, 2013. http://www.naturalnews.com/036328_Merck_mumps_vaccine_False_Claims_Act.html.

132 Odent MR, Culpin, EE, Kimmel, T. "Pertussis vaccine and asthma; is there a link?" Comment on *JAMA* 271 (March 23-30, 1994): 229-231.

133 Alm, J., J. Swartz, G. Lilja, A. Scheynius, and G. Pershagen. "Atopy in Children of Families with an Anthroposophic Lifestyle." *The Lancet* 353, no. 9163 (1999): 1485-488. doi:10.1016/S0140-6736(98)09344-1.

134 Shaheen, S. "Measles and Atopy in Guinea-Bissau." *The Lancet* 347, no. 9018 (June 19, 1996): 1792-796. doi:10.1016/S0140-6736(96)91617-7.

135 Kemp, Trudi, Neil Pearce, Penny Fitzharris, Julian Crane, and David Fergusson. "Is Infant Immunization a Risk Factor for Childhood Asthma or Allergy?" *Epidemiology* 8, no. 6 (November 1997): 678. doi:10.1097/00001648-199710000-00011.

136 Verrall M. "Pertussis vaccine linked to atopy." *Pulse.* May 1, 1999.

137 Donegan, Jayne L.M. "Whooping Cough: The Disease and the Vaccine. By Dr Jayne L M Donegan, June 2000." The Informed Parent (Magda Taylor), June 2000.

138 Long, G. H., A. T. Karanikas, E. T. Harvill, A. F. Read, and P. J. Hudson. "Acellular Pertussis Vaccination Facilitates Bordetella Parapertussis Infection in a Rodent Model of Bordetellosis." Proceedings of the Royal Society B: Biological Sciences 277, no. 1690 (June 26, 2010): 2017-025. doi:10.1098/rspb.2010.0010.

139 Noble, G.R., Bernier, R.H., Esber, E.C., Hardegree, M.C., et al. "Acellular and whole-cell pertussis vaccines in Japan: report of a visit by US scientists." *JAMA;* 257, no. 10 (1987): 1351-1356.

140 Van Buynder PG, Owen D, Vurdien JE, Andrews, NJ, Matthews RC, Miller E. Bordatella pertussis surveillance in England and Wales 1995-7. *Epidemiol. Inf.* 123, no. 3 (December 1999): 403-411.

141 Warfel, Jason M., Lindsey I. Zimmerman, and Todd J. Merkel. "Acellular Pertussis Vaccines Protect against Disease but Fail to Prevent Infection and Transmission in a Nonhuman Primate Model." Proceedings of the National Academy of Sciences, November 25, 2013.

142 Tsvernise, Sabrina. "Whooping Cough Study May Offer Clue on Surge." *New York Times*, November 25, 2013. Accessed November 28, 2013. http://www.nytimes.com/2013/11/26/health/study-finds-vaccinated-baboons-can-still-carry-whooping-cough.html?partner=rss&emc=rss.

143 Berg, J. M. "Neurological Complications of Pertussis Immunization." *BMJ* 2, no. 5087 (July 05, 1958): 24-27. doi:10.1136/bmj.2.5087.24.

144 Hilary Butler. "The Perilous Haemophilus or Is It.....pneumonia By Hilary Butler." The Perilous Haemophilus or Is It.....pneumonia By Hilary Butler. July 1996. http://www.whale.to/m/butler7.html.

145 Stephanie Cave and Deborah R. Mitchell. *What Your Doctor May Not Tell You about Children's Vaccinations.* New York: Warner Books, 2001. P. 137-144.

146 Juvenile Diabetes and Vaccination: New Evidence for a connection, National Vaccine Information Center.

147 Classen, B. "The Diabetes Epidemic Follows Hepatitis B Immunization Program." *New Zealand Medical Journal,* 109, no 195 (1996).

148 Classen DC, Classen JB. "The timing of pediatric immunization and the risk of insulin-dependent diabetes mellitus." *Infectious Diseases in Clinical Practice* 6 (1997): 449-54.

149 Dokheel TM. "An Epidemic of Childhood Diabetes in the United States." *Diabetes Care* 16 (1993): 1606-11.

150 Testimony to Congress, May 17, 1999, Classen, J. B. at http://www.whale.to/v/classen.html

151 Bokhari H. "Whooping cough in Pakistan: Bordetella pertussis vs Bordetella parapertussis in 2005-2009." *Scand J Infect Dis.* 43, no10 (October, 2011): 818-20.

152 Hegerle, N. Paris, A. Brun, D. Dore, G. Njamkepo, E. "Evolution of French Bordetella pertussis and Bordetella parapertussis isolates: increase of Bordetellae not expressing pertactin." *Clin Microbiol Infect.* 18, no. 9 (September 2012). DOI: 10.1111/j.1469-0691.2012.03925.x

153 Hambidge, M., and N. Krebs. "Zinc, Diarrhea, and Pneumonia." *The Journal of Pediatrics* 135, no. 6 (December 1999): 661-64. doi:10.1016/S0022-3476(99)70080-6.

154 Aiello, A., and E. Larson. "What Is the Evidence for a Causal Link between Hygiene and Infections?" *The Lancet Infectious Diseases* 2, no. 2 (February 2002): 103-10. doi:10.1016/S1473-3099(02)00184-6.

155 Vital Statistics of the United States 1937 Part I, U.S. Bureau of the Census, 1939, pp. 11-12; Vital Statistics of the United States 1938 Part I, U.S. Bureau of the Census, 1940, p. 12; Vital Statistics of the United States 1943 Part I, U.S. Bureau of the Census, 1945; Vital Statistics of the United States 1944 Part I, U.S. Bureau of the Census, 1946, p XXII-XXIII; Vital Statistics of the United States 1949 Part I, U.S. Public Health Service, 1951, p. XLIV; Vital Statistics of the United States 1960 Volume II – Mortality Part A, U.S. Department of Health, Education, and Welfare, 1963, p. 1-25; Vital Statistics of the United States 1967 Volume II – Mortality Part A, U.S. Department of Health, Education, and Welfare, 1969, p. 1-7; Vital Statistics of the United States 1976 Volume II – Mortality Part A, U.S. Department of Health and Human Services, 1980, p. 1-7; Vital Statistics of the United States 1987 Volume II – Mortality Part A, U.S. Department of Health and Human Services, 1990, p. 11; Vital Statistics of the United States 1992 Volume II – Mortality Part A, U.S. Department of Health and Human Services, 1996, p. 12; Historical Statistics of the United States – Colonial Times to 1970 Part 1, Bureau of the Census, p. 58.

156 Sienkiewicz D., Kulak W., Okurowska-Zawada B., and Paszko-Patej G. "Neurologic Adverse Events Following Vaccination." *Prog Health Sci.* 2, no. 1 (2012): 129-141.

157 Fisher, Barbara Loe. "Vaccine Contamination: Pig Virus DNA Found in Rotarix." National Vaccine Information Center (NVIC). April 4, 2010. Accessed September 29, 2013. http://www.nvic.org/nvic-vaccine-news/april-2010/vaccine-contamination-pig-virus-dna-found-in-rota.aspx.

158 NVIC.org. "49 Doses of 14 Vaccines Before the Age of 6? 69 Doses of 16 Vaccines Before the Age of 18? Before You Take the Risk, Find out What It Is." National Vaccine Information Center (NVIC). 2013. http://www.nvic.org/downloads/49-doses-posterb.aspx.

159 Janny Scott. "U.S. Slips Badly in Infant Mortality Fight, Panel Says." *Los Angeles Times* (Los Angeles) March 1, 1990, Collections ed., Trends sec.

160 McFarlane, Alex. "The Lancet IPad App: Articles in a New Light." INFANT DEATHS AFTER FOUR WEEKS : The Lancet. October 23, 1982. http://www.thelancet.com/journals/lancet/article/PIIS0140-6736(82)90892-3/fulltext.

161 Goldman, G.S."Relative trends in hospitalizations and mortality among infants by the number of vaccine doses and age, based on the Vaccine Adverse Event Reporting System (VAERS)," 1990-2010. *Hum Exp Toxicol* October 2012; 31(10): 1012-1021.

162 "Why Japan Stopped Using MMR." BBC News World Edition. BBC News Online, 8 Feb. 2002. Web.

163 Schubert J, Riley EJ, Tyler SA. "Combined effects in toxicology: A rapid systematic testing procedure: cadmium, mercury and lead." *Journal of Toxicology and Environmental Health.* 4 (1978): 763-776. - See more at: http://vactruth.com/2012/03/13/vaccines-human-animal-dna/#sthash.ekud27y0.dpuf

164 Sharpe, MA, Livingston, AD, and Baskin DS. "Thimerosal-Derived Ethylmercury Is a Mitochondrial Toxin in Human Astrocytes: Possible Role of Fenton Chemistry in the Oxidation and Breakage of mtDNA." *J Toxicol.* (2012): Article ID 373678. http://dx.doi.org/10.1155/2012/373678

165 "State of Health of Unvaccinated Children." *Survey Results.* Web. September 16, 2013. http://www.vaccineinjury.info/vaccinations-in-general/health-unvaccinated-children/survey-results-illnesses.html.

166 Glanz JM, Newcomer SR, Narwaney KJ, et al. "A population-based cohort study of undervaccination in 8 managed care organizations

across the United States". *JAMA Pediatr* 167, no 3 (March 1, 2013): 274-28.

167 Humphries, Suzanne, M.D., N.D. *"Vaccination Status and Health Outcomes among Homeschool Children."* December 23, 2012. Official Vaccinated vs Unvaccinated Study Finally Being Done, Jackson, MS, Salem Oregon.

168 Agmon-Levin, N., G.R. Hughes, and Y. Shoenfeld. "Autoimmune or Auto-inflammatory Syndrome Induced by Adjuvants (ASIA): Old Truths and a New Syndrome?" *Journal of Autoimmunity* 36, no. 1 (February 03, 2011): 4-8. doi:10.1016/j.jaut.2010.10.004.

169 Guillard, O. Fauconneau, G. Pineau, A. Marrauld, A. Bellocq, JP et al. "Aluminium overload after 5 years in skin biopsy following post-vaccination with subcutaneous pseudolymphoma." *J Trace Elem Med Biol.* 26, no. 4 (October 26, 2012).

170 Vera-Lastra, O. Medina, G. Del Pilar Cruz-Domingues, M. Jara, L. and Shoenfeld, Y. "Autoimmune/inflammatory syndrome induced by adjuvants (Shoenfeld's syndrome): clinical and immunological spectrum. Expert Reviews. *Expert Review of Clinical Immunology*, 9, no. 4 (April 2013): 361-373.

171 Shaw, C. A., and L. Tomljenovic. "Aluminum in the Central Nervous System (CNS): Toxicity in Humans and Animals, Vaccine Adjuvants, and Autoimmunity." Immunol. Res. 56, no. 2-3 (July 2013): 304-16. doi:10.1007/s12026-013-8403-1.

172 Asa, P. "Antibodies to Squalene in Gulf War Syndrome." *Experimental and Molecular Pathology* 68, no. 1 (February 2000): 55-64. doi:10.1006/exmp.1999.2295.

173 Statement in 2000 by Dr. Tom Verstraeten, CDC epidemiologist via the Freedom of Information Act. National Autism Association. From transcripts of the meeting (via FOIA). Received in an email dated June 28, 2006. http://www.thinktwice.com/aluminum.pdf

174 Aaby, P. "The Introduction of Diphtheria-tetanus-pertussis Vaccine and Child Mortality in Rural Guinea-Bissau: An Observational Study." International Journal of Epidemiology 33, no. 2 (April 01, 2004): 374-80. doi:10.1093/ije/dyh005.

175 Trapp GA, Minder, G.D., Zimmerman, R.L., Mastri, A.R. and Heston, L.L. "Aluminum levels in brain in Alzheimer's disease." *Biol Psychiatry.* 13, no 6 (December 13, 1978): 709-18.

176 Blank, M. Israeli, E. Shoenfeld, Y. "When APS (Hughes syndrome) met the autoimmune/inflammatory syndrome induced by adjuvants (ASIA)," *Lupus*, Vol 21, no.7 (June 2012): 711-714 doi: 10.1177/0961203312438115. http://lup.sagepub.com/content/21/7/711.long

177 Pequegnat, Brittany, Martin Sagermann, Moez Valliani, Michael Toh et al. "A Vaccine and Diagnostic Target for Clostridium Bolteae, an Autism-associated Bacterium." *Vaccine* 31, no. 26 (June 10, 2013): 2787-890.

178 Merck, Sharp & Dohme Corporation. M-M-R® II (MEASLES, MUMPS, and RUBELLA VIRUS VACCINE LIVE). Whitehouse Station: Merck &. http://www.fda.gov/downloads/BiologicsBloodVaccines/Vaccines/ApprovedProducts/UCM123789.pdf

179 Sin Hang Lee. "Topological conformational changes of human papillomavirus (HPV) DNA bound to an insoluble aluminum salt ~ A study by low temperature PCR." *Advances in Biological Chemistry*, 3 (2013): 76-85. ABC doi:10.4236/abc.2013.31010 Published Online February 2013.

180 Free Book by Hanan Polansky. "Microcompetition with Foreign DNA." Free Book by Hanan Polansky on Microcompetition with Foreign DNA. Accessed September 30, 2013. http://www.cbcd.net/Book.php.

181 NHS UK Government. "HPV Vaccine Side-effects." HPV Vaccine Side-effects. August 13, 2012. Accessed September 30, 2013. http://www.nhs.uk/Conditions/vaccinations/Pages/hpv-vaccine-cervarix-gardasil-side-effects.aspx.

182 Erickson, Norma. "HPV Vaccines and Idiopathic Thrombocytopenic Purpura." *SaneVax Inc*. SANEVax, Inc., 23 Apr. 2013. Web. June 16, 2013.

183 The Lead Vaccine Developer Comes Clean So She Can "Sleep At Night:" Gardasil and Ceravix Don't Work, Are Dangerous, and Weren't Tested. By Sarah Cain, The Liberty Becon. June 14, 2013.

184 Barr, J. et al. "Bacteriophage adhering to mucus provide a non–host-derived immunity,"

185 Barr, J. J., R. Auro, M. Furlan, and K. L. Whiteson. "Bacteriophage Adhering to Mucus Provide a Non–host-derived Immunity."

Proc Natl Acad Sci 110 (May 20, 2013): 10771-76. doi:10.1073/pnas.1305923110.

186 Moseman, E.A. Iannacone, M. Bosurgi, L. Tonti, E. Chevrier, N. et al. "B Cell Maintenance of Subcapsular Sinus Macrophages Protects against a Fatal Viral Infection Independent of Adaptive Immunity." Cell Press, 36, no. 3 (March 23, 2012). doi: 10.1016/j.immuni.2012.01.013

187 "Response to MDH Response to Testimony at Hearing and Comments Submitted." Jerri Johnson to Minnesota Department of Health OAH Rule Comments. July 24, 2013. Accessed October 28, 2013. http://www.health.state.mn.us/divs/idepc/immunize/immrule/comments/comment188.pdf.

188 Gallagher, Carolyn, and Melody Goodman. "Hepatitis B Vaccination of Male Neonates and Autism Diagnosis, NHIS 1997-2002." Journal of Toxicology and Environmental Health, Part A 73, no. 24 (January 2010): 1665-677. doi:10.1080/15287394.2010.519317.

189 James, S.j., William Slikker, Stepan Melnyk, Elizabeth New, Marta Pogribna, and Stefanie Jernigan. "Thimerosal Neurotoxicity Is Associated with Glutathione Depletion: Protection with Glutathione Precursors." NeuroToxicology 26, no. 1 (January 2005): 1-8. doi:10.1016/j.neuro.2004.07.012.

190 Zalups RK, et al. "Interactions between glutathione and mercury in the kidney, liver and blood." In: Chang, LW, ed. Toxicology of Metals. Boca Raton: CRC Press, 1996; 145-63.

191 Shenker BJ, et al. "Mercury-induced apoptosis in human lymphoid cells: evidence that the apoptotic pathway is mercurial species dependent." Environ Res (October, 2000): 84(2):89-99.

192 Hyman, MD, Mark. "Glutathione: The Mother of All Antioxidants." The Huffington Post. April 10, 2010. Accessed October 03, 2013. http://www.huffingtonpost.com/dr-mark-hyman/glutathione-the-mother-of_b_530494.html.

193 Associated Press. "Tylenol to Issue Warning Labels on Caps of Popular Pain Killer Alerting Users of Potentially Fatal Risks." NY Daily News. August 29, 2013. Accessed November 04, 2013. http://www.nydailynews.com/life-style/health/tylenol-issue-warnings-pill-bottles-article-1.1440915.

194 Becker, K. "Autism, Asthma, Inflammation, and the Hygiene Hypothesis." *Medical Hypotheses* 69, no. 4 (April 6, 2007): 731-40. doi:10.1016/j.mehy.2007.02.019.

195 Francisco Javier Gonzalez-Barcala, Sonia Pertega, Teresa Perez Castro, Manuel Sampedro, Juan Sanchez Lastres, Miguel Angel San Jose Gonzalez, Luis Bamonde, Luciano Garnelo, Luis Valdes, Jose-M Carreira, Jose Moure, and Angel Lopez Silvarrey "Exposure to paracetamol and asthma symptoms." *Eur J Public Health* 23. (2013): 706-710.

196 Schultz, S. T., H. S. Klonoff-Cohen, D. L. Wingard, N. A. Akshoomoff, et al. "Acetaminophen (paracetamol) Use, Measles-mumps-rubella Vaccination, and Autistic Disorder: The Results of a Parent Survey." *Autism* 12, no. 3 (May 29, 2008): 293-307. doi:10.1177/1362361307089518.

197 Brandlistuen, Ragnhild E., Eivind Ystrom, Irena Nulman, Gideon Koren, and Hedvig Nordeng. "Prenatal Paracetamol Exposure and Child Neurodevelopment: A Sibling-controlled Cohort Study." *Int. J. Epidemiol.*, October 24, 2013. doi:10.1093/ije/dyt183.

198 James SJ, Cutler P, Melnyk S, et al. "Metabolic biomarkers of increased oxidative stress and impaired methylation capacity in children with autism." *American Journal of Clinical Nutrition.* 80, no. 6 (December, 2004):1611–1617.

199 David Kirby, *Evidence of Harm: Mercury in Vaccines and the Autism Epidemic : A Medical Controversy.* New York: St. Martin's Press, 2005.

200 "Autism and Developmental Disabilities Monitoring (ADDM) Network." Centers for Disease Control and Prevention. March 29, 2012. Accessed December 16, 2012. http://www.cdc.gov/ncbddd/autism/addm.html.

201 "When 1 in 88 is Really 1 in 29." By Marcella. Vactruth.org. April 2012.

202 Tomljenovic, Lucija, and Christopher A. Shaw. "Do Aluminum Vaccine Adjuvants Contribute to the Rising Prevalence of Autism?" *Journal of Inorganic Biochemistry* 105, no. 11 (November 2011): 1489-499. doi:10.1016/j.jinorgbio.2011.08.008.

203 KIGGS Study. "State of Health of Unvaccinated Children." Survey Results Illnesses. Accessed September 30, 2013. http://www.vaccineinjury.info/vaccinations-in-general/health-unvaccinated-children/survey-results-illnesses.html.

204 Natasha Campbell-McBride,. *Gut and Psychology Syndrome: Natural Treatment for Autism, Dyspraxia, A.D.D., Dyslexia, A.D.H.D., Depression, Schizophrenia.* Cambridge, U.K.: Medinform Pub., 2010.

205 Wakefield, A., S. Murch, A. Anthony, and J. Linnell. "Ileal-lymphoid-nodular Hyperplasia, Non-specific Colitis, and Pervasive Developmental Disorder in Children." The Lancet 351, no. 9103 (February 28, 1998): 637-41. doi:10.1016/S0140-6736(97)11096-0.

206 Wakefield, Andrew, M.D. "The End Game." Health Freedom Expo. Renaissance Hotel, Chicago. June 16, 2012. Lecture.

207 "Vaccine Cases (UNPUBLISHED)." US Court of Federal Claims. Accessed September 30, 2013. http://www.uscfc.uscourts.gov/opinions_decisions_vaccine/Unpublished.

208 Attkisson, Sharyl. "Family to Receive $1.5M in First-Ever Vaccine-Autism Court Award." CBSNews. September 09, 2010. Accessed September 27, 2013. http://www.cbsnews.com/8301-31727_162-20015982-10391695.html.

209 Reid, Sue. "MMR: A Mother's Victory. The Vast Majority of Doctors Say There Is No Link between the Triple Jab and Autism, but Could an Italian Court Case Reignite This Controversial Debate?" Mail Online. June 15, 2012. Accessed September 27, 2013. http://www.dailymail.co.uk/news/article-2160054/MMR-A-mothers-victory-The-vast-majority-doctors-say-link-triple-jab-autism-Italian-court-case-reignite-controversial-debate.html.

210 "Whiteout Press." Courts Quietly Confirm MMR Vaccine Causes Autism. July 27, 2013. Accessed September 27, 2013. http://www.whiteoutpress.com/timeless/courts-quietly-confirm-mmr-vaccine-causes-autism/.

211 Singh, V. "Elevated Levels of Measles Antibodies in Children with Autism." *Pediatric Neurology* 28, no. 4 (April 2003): 292-94. doi:10.1016/S0887-8994(02)00627-6.

212 Geier, David, and Mark Geier. "An Evaluation of the Effects of Thimerosal on Neurodevelopmental Disorders Reported Following DTP and Hib Vaccines in Comparison to DTPH Vaccine in the United States." *Journal of Toxicology and Environmental Health Part A* 69, no. 15 (August 1, 2006): 1481-495. doi:10.1080/15287390500364556.

213 Young, Heather A., David A. Geier, and Mark R. Geier. "Thimerosal Exposure in Infants and Neurodevelopmental Disorders: An

Assessment of Computerized Medical Records in the Vaccine Safety Datalink." *Journal of the Neurological Sciences* 271, no. 1-2 (August 2008): 110-18. doi:10.1016/j.jns.2008.04.002.

214 Geier, David A., B. S. Hooker, J. K. Kern, and P. G. King. "A Two-phase Study Evaluating the Relationship between Thimerosal-containing Vaccine Administration and the Risk for an Autism Spectrum Disorder Diagnosis in the United States." *Transl. Neurodegener* 2, no. 1 (December 19, 2013): 25.

215 Geier DA, and Geier MR. "A comparative evaluation of the effects of MMR immunization and Mercury doses from thiomersal-containing childhood vaccines on the population prevalence of autism." *Med Sci Monit.* 10, no. 3 (March 2004): 133-9.

216 Young, Emma. "Gut Instincts: The Secrets of Your Second Brain." *New Scientisst,* December 17, 2012. doi:http://www.newscientist.com/article/mg21628951.900-gut-instincts-the-secrets-of-your-second-brain.html?full=true.

217 Gershon, Michael D. *The Second Brain.* New York:HarperCollins World, 1999.

218 A Contemporary View of Selected Subjects From the Pages of The New York Times, January 23, 1996. Printed in Themes of the Times: General Psychology, Fall 1996. Distributed Exclusively by Prentice-Hall Publishing Company. http://www.psyking.net/id36.htm.

219 Adam Hadhazy, "Think Twice: How the Gut's 'Second Brain' Influences Mood and Well-Being." *Scientific American,* February 12, 2010.

220 Yadov, V.K, Balagi, S. et al., "Pharmacological inhibition of gut-derived serotonin synthesis is a potential bone anabolic treatment for osteoporosis," *Nature Medicine* 16, 308–312. Published online 07 February 2010 Corrected online 17 February 2010.

221 Sandra Blakeslee, "Complex and Hidden Brain in Gut Makes Stomachaches and Butterflies," *New York Times,* January, 23, 1996.

222 G Clarke, S Grenham, P Scully, P Fitzgerald, R D Moloney, F Shanahan, T G Dinan and J F Cryan, Abstract for "The microbiome-gut-brain axis during early life regulates the hippocampal serotonergic system in a sex-dependent manner." *Molecular Psychiatry* June 12, 2012; doi:10.1038/mp.2012.77

223 Wakefield, Andrew, M.D. "The End Game." Lecture, Health Freedom Expo, Renaissance Hotel, Chicago. June 16, 2012. Lecture.

224 Karen E. Lasser, David U. Himmelstein, and Steffie Woolhandler. "Access to Care, Health Status, and Health Disparities in the United States and Canada: Results of a Cross-National Population-Based Survey." *Am J Public Health*, 96 (July 2006): 1300 - 1307.

225 Juster, F.T. National Institutes of Health, Health and Retirement Study, 2007, University of Michigan, Willis, R.J., Weir, D.R., to Ryff, C.D., Institute on Aging, University of Wisconsin; and Woodbury, R., National Bureau of Economic Research.

226 Devi, S, "Progress on childhood obesity patchy in the USA." *The Lancet*. 371, no 9607 (January 2008): 105-106.

227 U.S. Health in International Perspective: Shorter Lives, Poorer Health. The National Academies Press. 2013. http://www.nap. edu/catalog.php?record_id=13497

228 Rubenstein, Grace. "New Health Rankings: Of 17 Nations, U.S. Is Dead Last." The Atlantic. January 10, 2012. Accessed September 30, 2013. http://www.theatlantic.com/health/archive/2013/01/ new-health-rankings-of-17-nations-us-is-dead-last/267045/.

229 Stitt, Paul A. *Beating the Food Giants*. Natural Pr, 1982.

230 Clark LC, Combs GF, Jr., Turnbull BW, et al. "Effects of selenium supplementation for cancer prevention in patients with carcinoma of the skin. A randomized controlled trial." Nutritional Prevention of Cancer Study Group. *JAMA*. 276, no. 24 (December 25, 1996): 1957-63.

231 Ricciardolo FL, Rado V, Fabbri LM, Sterk PJ, Di Maria GU, Geppetti P. "Bronchoconstriction induced by citric acid inhalation in guinea pigs: role of tachycinins, bradykinin, and nitric oxide." 159 *Am J Respir Crit Care Med.* (1999): 557-62

232 Holma B, Lindegren M, Andersen JM. pH effects on ciliomotility and morphology of respiratory mucosa. *Arch Environ Health*. 32 (1977): 216-26.

233 Zhao J. Shimizu, T. Dobashi, K. Kawata, T. et al., "The Relationship between oxidative stress and acid stress in adult patients with mild asthma." *J Investig Allergol Clin Immunol* 18, no.1 (2008): 41-5.

234 Samsel, Anthony; Seneff, Stephanie. 2013. "Glyphosate's Suppression of Cytochrome P450 Enzymes and Amino Acid

Biosynthesis by the Gut Microbiome: Pathways to Modern Diseases." *Entropy* 15, no. 4 (April 18, 2013): 1416-1463.

235 Martino, Joe. "Aspartame Damages The Brain at Any Dose | Collective-Evolution." CollectiveEvolution RSS. October 06, 2013. Accessed October 27, 2013. http://www.collective-evolution. com/2012/10/06/aspartame-damages-the-brain-at-any-dose/.

236 Samsel, A. et al. "Glyphosate's Suppression of Cytochrome P450 Enzymes and Amino Acid Biosynthesis by the Gut Microbiome: Pathways to Modern Diseases."

237 "Stunning Corn Comparison: GMO versus NON GMO." Moms Across America. March 15, 2013. Accessed September 30, 2013. http://www.momsacrossamerica.com/ stunning_corn_comparison_gmo_versus_non_gmo.

238 Rates of Chronic Disease Expected to Rise Sharply. Clinical Laboratory News, July 2009.

239 Mayo Clinic. "Nearly 7 in 10 Americans are on prescription drugs." Mayo Clinic Proceedings June 19, 2013. Science Daily.

240 "Partnership to Fight Chronic Disease." Executive Summary: Partnership to Fight Chronic Disease. 2009. Accessed September 30, 2013. doi:http://www.fightchronicdisease.org/sites/fightchronicdisease.org/files/docs/PFCDAlmanac_ExecSum_updated81009.pdf

241 Abramov, Efrat, Iftach Dolev, Hilla Fogel, Giuseppe D. Ciccotosto, et al. "Amyloid-β as a Positive Endogenous Regulator of Release Probability at Hippocampal Synapses." *Nature Neuroscience* 12, no. 12 (December 12, 2009): 1567-576. doi:10.1038/nn.2433.

242 Richard R. Rubin, Yong Ma, Mark Peyrot, David G. Marrero Antidepressant Medicine Use and Risk of Developing Diabetes During the Diabetes Prevention Program and Diabetes Prevention Program Outcomes Study*Diabetes Care.* 33, no. 12 (December 2010): 2549–2551.. doi: 10.2337/dc10-1033

243 Campbell-McBride, *Gut and Psychology Syndrome.*

244 Hyppönen E, Läärä E, Reunanen A, Järvelin MR, Virtanen SM., Intake of vitamin D and risk of type 1 diabetes: a birth-cohort study., Lancet, 2001 Nov 3;358(9292):1500-3. Abstract].

245 Merlino, Linda A., Jeffrey Curtis, Ted R. Mikuls, and James R. Cerhan. "Vitamin D Intake Is Inversely Associated with Rheumatoid Arthritis: Results from the Iowa Women's Health

Study." Arthritis & Rheumatism 50, no. 1 (November 2004): 72-77. doi:10.1002/art.11434.

246 David Brownstein,. *Iodine: Why You Need It, Why You Can't Live without It.* West Bloomfield, MI: Medical Alternatives, 2009.

247 Vojdani A, Kharrazian D, Mukherjee PS. The Prevalence of Antibodies against Wheat and Milk Proteins in Blood Donors and Their Contribution to Neuroimmune Reactivities. *Nutrients.* 2014; 6(1):15-36.

248 Smith, Jeffrey M. "Institute for Responsible Technology." - Are Genetically Modified Foods a Gut-Wrenching Combination? November 2013. Accessed November 26, 2013. http://responsibletechnology.org/glutenintroduction.

249 Jerry Palmer, et al., "Identification of Autoantibody Negative Autoimmune Type 2 Diabetes Patients." *Diabetes Care.* 34, no.1 (January 2011): 168–173.

250 Braly, James, and Ron Hoggan. *Dangerous Grains: Why Gluten Cereal Grains May Be Hazardous to Your Health.* New York: Avery, 2002.

251 Challem, Jack, and Ronald E. Hunninghake. Stop Prediabetes Now: The Ultimate Plan to Lose Weight and Prevent Diabetes. Hoboken, NJ: John Wiley & Sons, 2007.

252 NotADoc.org. *About Chromium.* 2011. NEWtrition & You, a primer for life, Arkansas, Pocahontas.

253 Barton, Susan H., and Joseph A. Murray. "Celiac Disease and Autoimmunity in the Gut and Elsewhere." Gastroenterology Clinics of North America 37, no. 2 (June 2008): 411-28. doi:10.1016/j.gtc.2008.02.001.

254 Berer, Kerstin, Marsilius Mues, Michail Koutrolos, Zakeya Al Rasbi et al. "Commensal Microbiota and Myelin Autoantigen Cooperate to Trigger Autoimmune Demyelination." *Nature* 479, no. 7374 (November 26, 2011): 538-41. doi:10.1038/nature10554.

255 Jean-Claude Leunis, et al. "Increased serum IgA and IgM against LPS of enterobacteria in chronic fatigue syndrome (CFS): Indication for the involvement of gram-negative enterobacteria in the etiology of CFS and for the presence of an increased gut–intestinal permeability." *Journal of Affective Disorders.* 99, no. 1 (April 2007): 237 – 240.

256 Lundell, Dwight, M.D. "World Renown Heart Surgeon Speaks Out On What Really Causes Heart Disease." March 01, 2012. Accessed December 02, 2013. http://preventdisease.com/news/12/030112_World-Renown-Heart-Surgeon-Speaks-Out-On-What-Really-Causes-Heart-Disease.shtml.

257 Lundell, Dwight, and Todd R. Nordstrom. *The Cure for Heart Disease: Truth Will save a Nation.* Scottsdale, AZ: Heart Surgeon's Health Plan, 2007.

258 ibid. Robert J. Thiel, PhD. Naturopathy for the 21st Century. Whitman Publications. 2000.

259 Bracho, Gustavo, Enrique Varela, Rolando Fernández, and Barbara Ordaz. "Large-scale Application of Highly-diluted Bacteria for Leptospirosis Epidemic Control." *Homeopathy* 99, no. 3 (July 2010): 156-66.

260 Jensen, Bernard. The Chemistry of Man. 2nd ed. Escondido, CA: B. Jensen, 1983.

261 Gurudas. Flower Essences and Vibrational Healing. 3rd ed. San Rafael, CA: Cassandra Press, 1989. pp.30-31.

262 Jensen. B. *The Chemistry of Man.*

263 Romagnani, Sergio. "The Increased Prevalence of Allergy and the Hygiene Hypothesis: Missing Immune Deviation, Reduced Immune Suppression, or Both?" Immunology 112, no. 3 (July 2004): 352-63. doi:10.1111/j.1365-2567.2004.01925.x.

264 Randal Bollinger, R; Barbas, AS; Bush, EL; Lin, SS; Parker, W. "Biofilms in the large bowel suggest an apparent function of the human vermiform appendix." *Journal of Theoretical Biology.* 249 (2007): 826-831.

265 T. Olszak. An, D. Zeissis, S. Vera, M.P. et al., "Microbial exposure during early life has persistent effects on natural killer T cell function," *Science.* 336, no. 6080 (April 27, 2012) doi:10.1126/science.1219328, 2012.

266 Summers RW, Elliott DE, Urban JF, Thompson RA, Weinstock JV et al. "Trichuris suis therapy for active ulcerative colitis: a randomized controlled trial." *Gastroenterology.* 128 (2005): 825-832.

267 Weinstock JV, Elliott DE. "Helminths and the IBD hygiene hypothesis." *Inflamm Bowel Dis.* 15, no.1 (2009): 128-33.

268 Miller, S. "Old and New Rationales for Serum B12 and Folate Determinations." *Clinical Laboratory Sciences.* 6, no. 5 (1993): 272-274.

269 Fairbanks, V.F. "Iron in Medicine in Nutrition:185-213." In: *Modern Nutrition in Health and Disease*, 8th ed. M.E. Shils, J.A. Olson, and M.Shike, eds., Philadelphia, PA: Lea & Febinger, 1994, pp. 185-213.

270 Dr. Derry Interview with Mary Sholoman, July of 2000.

271 David Brownstein, David. *Overcoming Thyroid Disorders*. 2nd Ed. Medical Alternatives Press. 2002.

272 Fassa, Paul. "16 Magnesium Deficiency Symptoms – Signs of Low Magnesium Levels." Natural Society. April 1, 2013. Accessed September 30, 2013. http://naturalsociety.com/16-magnesium-deficiency-symptoms-signs-low-levels.

273 Berger, David, M.D., N.D. "Detoxification & Methylation." Talk About Curing Autism (TACA). March 15, 2013. Accessed October 23, 2013. http://www.tacanow.org/family-resources/detoxification-glutathione-autism/.

274 Otto H. Warburg, The Prime Cause and Prevention of Cancer accessed March 7, 2013

275 Raff, Neil. "August 2013 Dr. Neil Raff." Dr Neil Raff RSS. August 27, 2013. Accessed October 10, 2013. http://alternativeandcomplementarytherapies.org/2013/08/.

276 Wolff, Albert, "Eine medizinische verwendbarkeit des ozons." *Deutsche Medizinische Wochenschrift* (1915): 311-312, 1915.

277 Stoker, G. "The Surgical Uses Of Ozone." *The Lancet* 188, no. 4860 (1916): 712.

278 Guyot, René & C. -M. Roques, "L'eau de mer isotonique ozonisée pour le pansement des plaies de guerre. Un nouvel ozoneur." Comptes rendus des séances de la Société de biologie et de ses filiales 79 (1916): 289-290

279 Simard, S.W., Asay, A.K., Beiler, K.J., Bingham, M.A., Deslippe, J.R., He, X., Philip, L.J., Song, Y., Teste, F.P. . "Resource transfer between plants through ectomycorrhizal networks." – In: *Mycorrhizal Networks*. Edited by T. R. Horton. Springer, in review.

280 Bingham, M.A., and Simard, S.W. "Do mycorrhizal network benefits to survival and growth of interior Douglas-fir seedlings increase with soil moisture stress?" *Ecology and Evolution* 3, no. 1(2011): 306-316.

281 Jones MD, Twieg B, Ward V, Barker J, Durall DM, Simard SW. "Functional complementarity of Douglas-fir ectomycorrhizas for extracellularenzyme activity after wildfire or clearcut logging." *Functional Ecology*. 4: (2010): 1139-1151.

282 Alberda, C, Graf A, McCargar, L. "Malnutrition: etiology, consequences, and assessment of a patient at risk. *Best Pract Res Clin Gastroenterol* 20, no.3 (2006): 419–439.

283 Stroka, Knut. "Heart Catheter Film." Heart Attack. 2013. Accessed November 12, 2013. http://heartattacknew.com/heart-catheter-film/.

284 Thomas Cowan, M.D., Presentation at Wise Traditions Conference.

285 Stroka, K. "On the Genesis of Myocardial Ischemia." *Z Kardiol - Review* 93 (2004): 768-83. doi:10.1007/s00-392-004-0137-6.

286 Graham, Linda. "Bouncing Back: Rewiring Your Brain for Maximum Resilience." *Dharmaseed.org* (audio blog), November 7, 2013. Accessed November 24, 2013. http://dharmaseed.org/teacher/358/talk/21307/.

287 Davidson, Richard J., Ph.D. "Research in the News." Laboratory for Affective Neuroscience, UW-Madison Psychology Dept. http://psyphz.psych.wisc.edu/web/index.html.

288 Khosrotehrani, K. "Transfer of Fetal Cells With Multilineage Potential to Maternal Tissue." *JAMA: The Journal of the American Medical Association* 292, no. 1 (July 07, 2004): 75-80. doi:10.1001/jama.292.1.75.

289 Kara, Rina J., Ioannis Karakikes, Paola Bolli, Iwao Matsunaga, et al. "Fetal Cells Traffic to Injured Maternal Myocardium and Undergo Cardiac Differentiation." *Circ Res.* 110, no. 1 (January 6, 2012): 82-93. doi:22082491.

290 Koban M, Sita. L.V. Le, W.W. Hoffman, GE. "Sleep deprivation of rats: the hyperphagic response is real." *Sleep* 31(2006): 927–933.

291 Iliff, J.J., Wang, M., Liao, Y., Benjamin A. et al. "A Paravascular Pathway Facilitates CSF Flow Through the Brain Parenchyma and the Clearance of Interstitial Solutes, Including Amyloid β." *Science Translational Medicine*, 2012: DOI: 10.1126/scitranslmed.3003748

292 Clinton Ober, Stephen T. Sinatra, and Martin Zucker. *Earthing: The Most Important Health Discovery Ever?* Laguna Beach, CA: Basic Health Publications, 2010.

293 McDougall, Christopher. *Born to Run: A Hidden Tribe, Superathletes, and the Greatest Race the World Has Never Seen.* New York: Alfred A. Knopf, 2009

294 Young, C. "The Truth About Hair and Why Indians Would Keep Their Hair Long -- Science of the Spirit -- Sott.net." Signs of the Times. September 08, 2011. Accessed October 20, 2013. doi:SOTT.net.

295 Kunzig, Robert. "The Biology of . . . Hair Zeroing in on the Molecular Switches That Regulate Hair Growth." Discover Magazine. February 01, 2002. Accessed October 20, 2013. http://discovermagazine.com/2002/feb/featbiology.

296 *From the Heart of the World: Elder Brother's Warning.* Directed by Alan Ereira. Performed by The Kogi Mamos. England: British Broadcasting Corporation, 1989. Documentary.

297 Robert K.G. Temple, *The Sirius Mystery: New Scientific Evidence of Alien Contact 5,000 Years Ago.* Rochester, VT: Destiny Books, 1998.

298 Lawrence, L. George. "Interstellar Communications Signals." *Journal of Borderland Research* 29, no. 4 (July/August 1973).

299 Bell, Robert Scott. "Spender-Jacklin-Abbot." The Robert Scott Bell Show. Natural News Radio. Aug. 1, 2013. Radio.

300 Hampson, Aidan J., Julius Axelrod, and Maurizio Grimaldi. Cannabinoids as Antioxidants and Neuroprotectants. US Patent 6630507, filed February 02, 2001, and issued October 07, 2003.

301 Rudolph Ballentine, Rudolph. *Diet and Nutrition a Holistic Approach.* Honesdale, Pa: Himalayan International Institute, 1979

302 Beddoe, *Biologic Ionization as applied to human nutrition,*

303 Beddoe, *Biologic Ionization as applied to human nutrition,* p. 30.

304 Henry Lindlahr, *Nature Cure: Philosophy and Practice Based on the Unity of Disease and Cure.* Chicago: Nature Cure Pub., 1922.

305 "Thomas Szasz on Freedom and Psychotherapy." Interview by Randall C. Wyatt. Psychotherapy.net/interview. Psychotherapy. net, Dec. 2000. Web. 24 Sept. 2013. <http://www.psychotherapy. net/interview/thomas-szasz>.

306 Seewer, John. "Ohio Amish Girl Won't Be Forced to Renew Chemo." *U-T San Diego.* Associated Press, 6 Dec. 2013. Web. 09 Dec. 2013.

307 Glanzer, Kaitlin. "Protest Planned to Fight Hospital's 'Kidnapping' of West Hartford Girl [Updated]." *West Hartford Patch.* N.p., 2 Dec. 2013. Web. 09 Dec. 2013.

308 Gumpert, David. "When the State Becomes the Parent of Force." *The Complete Patient.* N.p., 4 Dec. 2013. Web. 09 Dec. 2013.

309 Nestor, Moritz. "Inventor of ADHD: "ADHD Is a Fictitious Disease."" *Current Concerns* 9 (2012).

310 Rovet, Richard, RN, BSN, B-C (USAF Ret). "ARPR - Captain Richard Rovet, RN - Our Soldiers Should Have the Same Vaccine Rights." YouTube. July 09, 2010. Accessed October 15, 2013. http://www.youtube.com/watch?v=BcpSsZeJ-1M.

311 Kiddie, Joy Y., Margaret D. Weiss, David D. Kitts, Ryna Levy-Milne, and Michael B. Wasdell. "Nutritional Status of Children with Attention Deficit Hyperactivity Disorder: A Pilot Study." *International Journal of Pediatrics* 2010 (June 28, 2010): 1-7. doi:10.1155/2010/767318.

312 Lau, K. "Synergistic Interactions between Commonly Used Food Additives in a Developmental Neurotoxicity Test." *Toxicological Sciences* 90, no. 1 (March 30, 2005): 178-87. doi:10.1093/toxsci/kfj073.

313 Lafferman, J., and E. Silbergeld. "Erythrosin B Inhibits Dopamine Transport in Rat Caudate Synaptosomes." *Science* 205, no. 4404 (July 27, 1979): 410-12. doi:10.1126/science.451609.

314 Pelsser, Lidy M., Klaas Frankena, Jan Toorman, Huub F. Savelkoul, et al. "Effects of a Restricted Elimination Diet on the Behaviour of Children with Attention-deficit Hyperactivity Disorder (INCA Study): A Randomised Controlled Trial." *The Lancet* 377, no. 9764 (February 2011): 494-503. doi:10.1016/S0140-6736(10)62227-1.

315 Sears, William. *The N.D.D. Book: How Nutrition Deficit Disorder Affects Your Child's Learning, Behavior, and Health, and What You Can Do about It--without Drugs.* New York: Little, Brown, 2009.

316 Hancock, Graham. "Graham Hancock - The War on Consciousness @ TEDxWhitechapel." YouTube. YouTube, 14 Mar. 2013. Web. 27 Sept. 2013.

317 Robert Levenson, Ph.D., professor, psychology, University of California, Berkeley; Paul Zak, Ph.D., chairman and professor, economics, and founding director, Center for Neuroeconomics Studies, Claremont Graduate University, Claremont, Calif. *Emotion* Oct. 7, 2013.

318 Ms. Harry's comments in the International Forum on Globalization Teach-in held in New York City in February 2001 were based on her recent article, *Biopiracy and Globalization: Indigenous Peoples Face a New Wave of Colonialism*, published in the magazine Splice, January/April 2001 Volume 7 Issues 2 & 3

319 Bruce H. Lipton, *The Biology of Belief.* Memphis, TN: Spirit 2000. 2003.

320 Bruce H. Lipton, *The Biology of Perception, The Psychology of Change.* Bruce H. Lipton. Mountain Love Productions, 2001, DVD.

321 El-Osta, A., D. Brasacchio, D. Yao, A. Pocai, et al. "Transient High Glucose Causes Persistent Epigenetic Changes and Altered Gene Expression during Subsequent Normoglycemia." *Journal of Experimental Medicine* 205, no. 11 (September 06, 2008): 2683. doi:10.1084/jem.20081188092608c.

322 Shaheen, S. "Measles and Atopy in Guinea-Bissau." *The Lancet* 347, no. 9018 (June 19, 1996): 1792-796. doi:10.1016/S0140-6736(96)91617-7.

323 Freeman, Elliot. "Scientists: New GMO Wheat May 'silence' Vital Human Genes Special." Scientists: New GMO Wheat May 'silence' Vital Human Genes (Includes Interview). October 9, 2012. Accessed May 30, 2013. http://www.digitaljournal.com/article/332822.

324 Gariaev P.P., Kaznacheev V.P., Vasiliev A.A., berezin A.A. Soliton-holographic genome with a collectively-symmetrical genetic code. Preprint. SO Acad. of Medical Sciences. Inst. of clinic and expert. medicine. (1990) p.50.

325 Gregg Braden, *The Spontaneous Healing of Belief: Shattering the Paradigm of False Limits.* Carlsbad, CA: Hay House, 2008. P. 131.

326 Fang, F., M.D., K. Fall, M.D., M. A. Mittleman, M.D. P. Sparen, M.D. et al. "Immediate Risk of Suicide and Cardiovascular Death After a Prostate Cancer Diagnosis: Cohort Study in the United States." *NEJM* 366 (April 5, 2012): 1310-18. doi:10.1056/NEJMoa1110307.

327 Brodersen, J. Siersma, V.D. "Long-term psychosocial consequences of false-positive screening mammography." *Ann Fam Med.* (Mar-Apr, 2013): 11(2):106-15.

328 Gariaev, P. P., and A. A. Berezin. "Soliton-holographic Genome with a Collectively-symmetrical Genetic Code." In *SO Acad. of Medical Sciences,* by V. P. Kaznacheev, *50.* Inst. of Clinic and Expert Medicine, 1990.

329 Gariaev, P. P. Wave genome, Public profit. 1994. Moscow. 279 pages [in Russian].

330 Fosar, Grazyna, and Framz Bludorf. "Scientist Proves DNA Can Be Reprogrammed by Words and Frequencies." My Natures Medicinecom. August 5, 2013. http://mynaturesmedicine.com/2013/08/05/scientist-proves-dna-can-be-reprogrammed-by-words-and-frequencies/.

331 Brennan, Barbara Ann. Hands of Light: A Guide to Healing through the Human Energy Field. Toronto: Bantam Books, 1987.

332 Gonit, Sora. "E=mc^2 : Equation of Life and Death. March 7, 2013. http://gonitsora.com/emc2-equation-of-life-and-death/.

333 Robinson, Andrew. The Last Man Who Knew Everything: Thomas Young, the Anonymous Genius Who Proved Newton Wrong, and Deciphered the Rosetta Stone, among Other Surprising Feats. New York: Plume, 2007.

334 Alberto Peruzzo, Peter Shadbolt, Nicolas Brunner, Sandu Popescu, and Jeremy L. O'Brien. A Quantum Delayed-Choice Experiment. Science, 2012; 338 (6107): 634-637 DOI: 10.1126/science.1126719.

335 Tiller, William A. "How the Power of Intention Alters Matter with Dr. William A. Tiller - StumbleUpon." Spiritofmaat.com. http://www.stumbleupon.com/su/2StYxR

336 Monk, Michael. "The Collective Imagination." Interview.

337 Bruyere, Rosalyn L. Wheels of Light: Chakras, Auras, and the Healing Energy of the Body. New York: Fireside Book, 1994.

338 Lo, Shui Lin, Ph.D. "Quantum Healing with Dr. Lo." YouTube. January 15, 2007. Accessed November 30, 2013. https://www.youtube.com/watch?v=uG8pGSxNrZ8.

339 Sereda, David, writer. "Quantum Communication." In Quantum Communication. Coast to Coast Am with George Noory. August 8, 2009.

340 Vitale, Joe, and Len Haleakalā. Hew. Zero Limits: The Secret Hawaiian System for Wealth, Health, Peace, and More. Hoboken, NJ: Wiley, 2007.

341 Katz, Micahel. Wisdom of the Gemstone Guardians. p. 18.

342 Taylor, Eldon. *I Believe: When What You Believe Matters!* London: Hay House, 2013.

343 Kamp, Jurriaan. "A Change of Heart Changes Everything." Ode Magazine, no. 24 (June 2005).

344 Kremer, H. Ironson, G. Kaplan, L. Stuetzle, R. and Fletcher, M.A. "Compassionate Love as a Predictor of Reduced HIV Disease Progression and Transmission Risk," *Evidence-Based Complementary and Alternative Medicine*, (2013) Article ID 819021. 2013. doi:10.1155/2013/819021

345 "Rupert Sheldrake - The Science Delusion BANNED TED TALK." YouTube. March 15, 2013. Accessed September 15, 2013. https://www.youtube.com/watch?v=JKHUaNAxsTg.

346 Hancock, Graham. "Graham Hancock - The War on Consciousness @ TEDxWhitechapel." YouTube. 14 Mar. 2013. Assessed September 27, 2013.

347 Maddox, General. "The Hegelian Dialectic and Its Use in Controlling Modern Society." Real News Australia. April 8, 2013. http://realnewsaustralia.com/2013/08/09/the-hegelian-dialectic-and-its-use-in-controlling-modern-society/.

348 South v. Maryland, 59 U.S. (How.) 396, 15 L.Ed.433 (1856)

349 Bowers v. Devito, 686 F.2d 616 (7th Cir. 1982)

350 Hawkins, David R. Power vs. Force: The Hidden Determinants of Human Behavior. Carlsbad, CA: Hay House, 2002.

351 Carus, Paul. Karma: A Story of Buddhist Ethics. Chicago [u.a.: Open Court Pub. [u.a., 1903.

352 Printz, C. "Radiation Treatment Generates Therapy-resistant Cancer Stem Cells from Less Aggressive Breast Cancer Cells." Cancer 118, no. 13 (July 01, 2012): 3225. doi:10.1002/cncr.27701.

353 Ruocco, Margaret. From the Mouth of Babes. 2010. True story re-layed by author's sister from her son Chase, age nine. Milwaukee.

354 "Psychic & Awakened Children." Millennium Education. N.p., n.d. Web.

355 Dispenza, Joe. Evolve Your Brain: The Science of Changing Your Mind. Dearfield, FL: Health Communications, 2007.

356 "David Lynch Foundation." Meditation in Schools (Quiet Time Program) -. http://www.davidlynchfoundation.org/schools.html

357 Katz, Michael. Wisdom of the Gemstone Guardians. pp. 25-26.

358 ibid. Gurudas. p. 31

359 ibid. Gurudas. p. 86

360 Talbot, Michael. The Holographic Universe. New York: HarperCollins, 1991.

361 "The Holographic Universe - 1 of 5 - Quantum Physics." YouTube. YouTube, 19 Jan. 2013. Web. 15 Sept. 2013.

362 Marcus, Aurelius, and Gregory Hays. Meditations. New York: Modern Library, 2002.

363 Michael Newton. Journey of Souls: Case Studies of Life between Lives. St. Paul, MN: Llewellyn, 1994.

364 McCants, Glynis. *Love by the Numbers: How to Find Great Love or Reignite the Love You Have through the Power of Numerology.* Naperville, IL: Sourcebooks Casablanca, 2009.

365 Schroeder, Carl J. "New Earth Light." : Surviving the Twin Soul. August 24, 2011. http://newearthlight.blogspot.com/2011/08/surviving-twin-flame.html.

366 Fenn, Celia. "Uniting with Your Twin Flame." Uniting with Your Twin Flame. http://www.starchildglobal.com/starchild/twin-flame2.html.

367 Stevenson, Ian. Children Who Remember Past Lives: A Question of Reincarnation. McFarland, 2000.

368 Eshowsky, Myron. *Peace with Cancer: Shamanism as a Spiritual Approach to Healing.* Madison, WI: Shoshana Publications, 2009.

369 Snstein2nh329. "The Amazing Power Of Crystal Grids." Scribd. N.p., 2007. Accessed July 2, 2013. http://www.scribd.com/doc/7778924/The-Amazing-Power-Of-Crystal-Grids-.

370 Hagelin J.S. et al. "Effects of group practice of the Transcendental Meditation program on preventing violent crime in Washington, DC: Results of the National Demonstration Project. June-July 1993." *Social Indicators Research* 47 (1999): 153-201.

371 David W. Orme-Johnson, Charles N. Alexander, John L. Davies, Howard M. Chandler, and Wallace E. Larimore. "International Peace Project in the Middle East: The Effects of the Maharishi Technology of the Unified Field." *Journal of Conflict Resolution* 32 (December, 1988): 776-812, doi:10.1177/0022002788032004009

372 Hagelin, John, Ph.D. *The Power of the Collective.* Proceedings of Shift: At the Frontiers of Consciousness, IONS Regional Conference, Tucson. Vol. 15. N.p.: Istpp.org, 2007. 16-20. Http://istpp.org/pdf/Shift-PoweroftheCollective.pdf.

373 Lamb, Gregory M. "Study Highlights Difficulty of Isolating Effect of Prayer on Patients." *Christian Science Monitor.* April 3, 2006.

374 Smith, Jack. "The Square Root of 1% of the Population Unified in Any Way May Be the Greatest Discovery in the History of Science." Los Angeles Times (Los Angeles), May 8, 1986.

375 "The Maharishi Effect." Dubrovnik Peace Project. October 15, 2011. Accessed September 16, 2013. http://www.dubrovnik-peace-project.org/sci/maharishi_effect.htm.

376 Monk, Michael. "The Collective Imagination." Interview by Lisa M. Harrison, Bob Wright, and Brian Kelly. *Blogtalkradio.com*. 5D Media Network. 1 Oct. 2013. Radio.

377 ibid David R. Hawkins. *Power vs. Force: The Hidden Determinants of Human Behavior.*

378 ibid. Gurudas. *Flower Essences.*

379 Rosen, Marc S. and Williams, L. *The Research Status of Applied Kinesiology, Part II: An Annotated Bibliography of Applied Kinesiological Research.* In: A.K. Review, Vol. 1. No. 2: 34-47, 1991.

380 Thiel, Robert J. "Chronic Fatigue Assessment and Intervention: The Result of 101 Cases." *ANMA & AANC J.* 1, no 3. (1996): 17-19.

381 Thiel, Robert J. "Natural Interventions for People with Fibromyalgia." *ANMA Monitor.* 2, no. 2 (1998): 6-8.

382 Viktoras P. Kulvinskas, *Survival into the 21st Century: Planetary Healers Manual.* Woodstock Valley, Ct.: 21st Century Publications, 1975.

383 Aldridge, D., et al. "Where am I? Music therapy Applied to Coma Patients." *J Roy Soc Med.* 83 (1990): 345-346.

384 Harding, Suzanne. "More Noise or Sound Theory?" Alternative and Complementary Therapies 5, no. 3 (1999): 164-74. doi:10.1089/act.1999.5.164.

385 Oster, Gerald. "Auditory Beats in the Brain." *Scientific American.* October, 1973.

386 Swami Krishnananda, *The Māndūkya Upaniṣad: An Exposition.* Shivanandanagar: Divine Life Society, 1977.

387 Yogendra Nath Yogi. "Yogendra Nath Yogi." Yogendra Nath Yogi. May 16, 2011. Accessed September 30, 2013. http://yogendranath-yogi.webs.com/apps/blog/entries/show/7062236-om-in-the-upanishads-bhagavad-gita-and-yoga-sutras.

388 Easwaran, Eknath. *The Upanishads: A Classic of Indian Spirituality.* 2nd ed. Nilgiri Press, 2007.

389 SuperHealth. "The Causes of Addiction from a Yogic Perspective." Kundalini Yoga as Taught by Yogi Bahjan. Accessed December 09, 2013. http://www.3ho.org/3ho-lifestyle/health-and-healing/kundalini-yoga-and-use-recreational-drugs/causes-addiction-yogic.

390 Telles, Shirley, R. Nagarathna, and H.R. Nagendra. "Physiological Measures of Right Nostril Breathing." The Journal of Alternative

and Complementary Medicine 2, no. 4 (1996): 479-84. doi:10.1089/acm.1996.2.479.

391 Swami Ramdev. Chapater: *Hatha yoga and Satkarma.* In: Yoga sadhana and Yog chikitsa rahasya. Divya prakashan. Diva yog mandir (trust). Kanakhal. Haridwar. (2004): 114-20.

392 Malhotra, V, Dhungle, K.U., J. Ganga. "Does the Effect of Pranayama Differ in Yoga Practitioner and naïve? *Journal of Clinical and Diagnostic Research.* 4, no.6 (December 2010): 3503-3506.

393 Bhajan, Yogi, Ph.D. *The Aquarian Teacher - KRI International Kundalini Yoga Teacher Training Level I Yoga Manual - Part Nine, Sets and Meditations.* 3rd ed. Kundalini Research Institute, 2005.

394 Yogananda. Autobiography of a Yogi. Los Angeles: Self-Realization Fellowship, 2010.

395 Yogananda, Paramahansa. *The Yoga of Jesus: Understanding the Hidden Teachings of the Gospels : Selections from the Writings of Paramahansa Yogananda.* Los Angeles: Self-Realization Fellowship, 2007.

396 Yogandanda, P. *The Yoga of Jesus*

397 Ravi Singh, *Kundalini Yoga.* New York: White Lion, 2000.

398 Sabrina Mesko, Sbrina. *Healing Moudras.* New York: Ballantine Wellspring, 2000.

399 Gaynor, Mitchell L. *Sounds of Healing: A Physician Reveals the Therapeutic Power of Sound, Voice, and Music.* New York: Broadway, 1999.

400 Robert Lawrence Friedman. *The Healing Power of the Drum.* Reno, NV: White Cliffs Media, 2000.

401 Michael Winkelman. *Shamanism: The Neural Ecology of Consciousness and Healing.* Westport, CT: Bergin & Garvey, 2000.

402 Minchin, Tim. "OCCASIONAL ADDRESS." *Tim Minchin.com News and Blog* (web log), September 25, 2013. Accessed October 14, 2013. http://www.timminchin.com/2013/09/25/occasional-address/.

403 Maharshi, Ramana. "Happiness." September 6, 2000. Accessed October 12, 2013. http://maharshi.bizland.com/happiness.htm.

404 Kaleem Gill, MD. "Fight or Flight and Eat? Stress Can Contribute to Weight Gain." *The Blade (Toledo),* September 6, 2013.

405 Mark, David, MA. "The Metabolic Power of Pleasure." *Psychologyofeating.com/metabolic-power-pleasure.* N.p., 5 June 2013. Web

406 Calabrese, Adrian. *Sacred Signs: Hear, See & Believe Messages from the Universe.* Woodbury, MN: Llewellyn, 2006.

407 E.W. Dubstova, *Clinical Studies with Bee Products for Therapy of Some Nutritional Diseases*. Moscow: Central Moscow Institute of Gastroenterology, 2009. pp 1-38.

408 Sandra Ingerman. *Shamanic Journeying: A Beginner's Guide*. Boulder, CO: Sounds True, 2008.

409 Ingerman, S. *Shamanic Journeying*.

410 *The Shadow Effect: Illuminating the Hidden Power of Your True Self*. Directed by Debbie Ford. Performed by Debbie Ford, Deepak Chopra, James Van Praagh, Mark Victor Hansen, Marianne Williamson. HarperOne, 2010. DVD.

411 Andrew J. Armour and Jeffrey L. Ardell. *Neurocardiology*. New York: Oxford University Press, 1994.

412 McCraty, Rollin, Ph.D. "The Energetic Heat: Bioelectrical Interactions Within and Between People." Institute of HeartMath. Accessed June 2, 2012. http://www.heartmath.org/free-services/articles-of-the-heart/energetic-heart-is-unfolding.html.

413 Mimi Guarneri, *The Heart Speaks: A Cardiologist Reveals the Secret Language of Healing*. New York: Simon & Schuster, 2006.

414 McCraty, R. Ph.D., Atkinson, M. Tomasino, D. B.A., and Tiller, W. A. Ph.D. "The Electricity of Touch: Detection and Measurement of Cardiac Energy Exchange Between People, In: Karl H. Pribram, ed. *Brain and Values: Is a Biological Science of Values Possible*. Mahwah, NJ: Lawrence Erlbaum Associates, (1998): 359-379.

415 Braden, Gregg. "Gregg Braden on Consciousness." *YouTube*. YouTube, 19 Feb. 2009. Web. 17 Oct. 2013.

416 An excerpt taken from "A Conversation With Eckhart Tolle And Deepak Chopra" Video can also be found at http://youtu.be/q5J4HbmVfvA ~ at Chopra Center.

417 Carey A. Reams, *Choose! Life or Death: The Reams Biological Theory of Ionization*. Harrison, AR: New Leaf, 1978.

418 Vachon, Marc, and Amy Vachon. *Equally Shared Parenting: Rewriting the Rules for a New Generation of Parents*. New York: Penguin Group, 2010.

419 *The Secret Life of Plants*. Directed by Walon Green and Christopher Bird. By Peter Tompkins. Performed by Ruby Crystal, John Ashley Hamilton. Paramount Pictures, 1979. Documentary.

420 *What Plants Talk About*. Performed by JC Cahill. Merit Motion Pictures Production/Nature and WNET for PBS, 2013. DVD.

421 Gurian-Sherman, Doug. Failure to Yield Evaluating the Performance of Genetically Engineered Crops. Issue brief. Cambridge, U.K.: Union of Concerned Scientists, 2009.

422 deGrassi, Aaron. "Monsanto's showcase project in Africa fails." *New Scientist.* 181, no. 2433 (February 7, 2004).

423 Gassmann AJ, Petzold-Maxwell JL, Keweshan RS, and Dunbar MW. "Field-Evolved Resistance to Bt Maize by Western Corn Rootworm." PLoS ONE 6, no 7 (2011): e22629. doi:10.1371/journal.pone.0022629

424 Philpott, Tom. "Attack of the Monsanto Superinsects." MotherJones. August 30, 2011. Accessed September 20, 2013. http://www.motherjones.com/tom-philpott/2011/08/monsanto-gm-super-insects.

425 Benbrook, Charles M. "Impacts of Genetically Engineered Crops on Pesticide Use in the U.S. -- the First Sixteen Years." *Environmental Sciences Europe* 24.24 (2012): 1-13.

426 Heinemann, J.A. Massaro, M. Coray, D.S. Aanon Agapito-Tenfen and Wen, J. S. "Sustainability and Innovation in Staple Crop Production in the US Midwest." Sustainability and Innovation in Staple Crop Production in the US Midwest. Taylor and Francis. June 14, 2013. Accessed September 23 2013.

427 Kessler, Rebecca. "Superbug Hideout: Finding MRSA in U.S. Wastewater Treatment Plants." *Environ Health Perspect.* A437 no. 120.11 (November, 2012).

428 VERNON HUGH BOWMAN v. MONSANTO CO., ET AL.,. 11-796. Supreme Court of the United States. December 10, 2012.

429 Hopwood, Jennifer, Mace Vaughn, Matthew Shepherd, David Biddinger, Eric Mader, Scott H. Black, and Celeste Mazzacano. "The Xerces Society for Invertebrate Conservation." Review of A Review of Research into the Effects of Neonicotinoid Insecticides on Bees, with Recommendations for Action. The Xerces Society for Invertebrate Conservation, 2012. 2012. http://ento.psu.edu/publications/are-neonicotinoids-killing-bees.

430 Pettis JS, Lichtenberg EM, Andree M, Stitzinger J, Rose R, et al. "Crop Pollination Exposes Honey Bees to Pesticides Which Alters Their Susceptibility to the Gut Pathogen *Nosema ceranae.*" *PLoS ONE* 8, no 7. (2013): e70182. doi:10.1371/journal.pone.0070182

431 Netherwood, Trudy, Susana M. Martín-Orúe, Anthony G. O'Donnell, and Sally Gockling. "Assessing the Survival of Transgenic Plant DNA in the Human Gastrointestinal Tract." *Nature Biotechnology* 22, no 2 (2004): 204-09.

432 BBC News. "Scientists given Cloning Go-ahead." *BBC News,* November 08, 2004. Accessed October 15, 2013. http://news.bbc. co.uk/2/hi/health/3554474.stm.

433 Ji, Sayer. "Biotech's Dark Promise: Involuntary Cannibalism for All - Page 2." Biotech's Dark Promise: Involuntary Cannibalism for All - Page 2. October 15, 2013. Accessed October 15, 2013. http://www.greenmedinfo.com/blog/ biotechs-dark-promise-involuntary-cannabilism-all-1?page=2.

434 VandenDolder, Tess. "Corporate Inventor of GMOs Protected in Congressional Bill Angering Consumer Advocates." InTheCapital. InTheCaptial, April 1, 2013. Accessed September 20, 2013. http:// inthecapital.streetwise.co/2013/04/01/congressional-corporate-pandering-upsets-food-safety-advocates/.

435 Alex Renton, "India's Hidden Climate Change Catastrophe Over the past Decade, as Crops Have Failed Year after Year, 200,000 Farmers Have Killed Themselves." *The Independent,* London, January 2, 2011.

436 Mayfield, Elanor. "Design Dilemma: The Debate over Using Placebos in Cancer Clinical Trials." NCI Cancer Bulletin for May 3, 2011. May 03, 2011. Accessed October 20, 2013. http://www.cancer.gov/ncicancerbulletin/050311/page7.

437 Gøtzsche, Peter C., M.D. "Deadly Medicines and Organised Crime - Peter Gøtzsche." Jeffrey Dach M.D. October 3, 2013. Accessed December 09, 2013. http://jeffreydachmd.com/2013/12/ modern-medicine-organized-crime-peter-gotzsche/.

438 Gonzalez, Nicholas James. *What Went Wrong. the Truth behind the Clinical Trial of the Enzyme Treatment of Cancer.* New York, NY, USA: New Spring Press, 2012.

439 Siriporn Thongprakaisang, Apinya Thiantanawat, Nuchanart Rangkadilok, Tawit Suriyo, Jutamaad Satayavivad. "Glyphosate induces human breast cancer cells growth via estrogen receptors." *Food Chem Toxicol.* June 8, 2013.

440 Tiller, William A. Ph.D. "Psychoenergetic Science Applied to the Mind-Body Concept." White Paper. September 2010.

441 "Food Swap Network." Food Swap Network. 2013. Accessed October 19, 2013. http://www.foodswapnetwork.com/.

442 Cahn, Edgar S. *No More Throw-away People: The Co-production Imperative.* Washington, D.C.: Essential, 2000.

443 Fraser, Nathaniel Anton. *As King: A Simple Guide to Autonomous Living.* Livefree.fm, 2001. http://www.reallyweirdstuff.com/AsKing-FreeDownLoad.pdf.

444 Blanchard, Beverly. "The Law of Assumption." Waking Times. October 28, 2013. Accessed October 27, 2013. http://www.waking-times.com/2013/10/26/law-assumption/.

445 Emoto, Masaru. *The Hidden Messages in Water.* Hillsboro, Or.: Beyond Words Pub., 2004.

446 *Water, the Great Mystery.* Directed by Saida Medvedeva. USA and Canada: Intention Media Inc.

447 Emoto, Marasu, and Konstantin Korotkov, Ph.D. *Baikal Water Ceremony, August 3, 2008.* Report. July 9, 2012. http://korotkov.org/baikal-water-ceremony/#more-756.

448 Hildebrandt, Sybille. "Soil Bacteria Can Clean Your Drinking Water." Sciencenordic.com. March 8, 2013. http://sciencenordic.com/soil-bacteria-can-clean-your-drinking-water.

449 Deutsch, Claudia. "A Single Source for Clean Water and Fuel." *New Scientist* - Tech. April 13, 2011. Accessed October 01, 2013. http://www.newscientist.com/article/mg21028075.300-a-single-source-for-clean-water-and-fuel.html.

450 Leonard G. Horowitz, Ph.D., and Joseph Puleo, N.D. *Healing Codes for the Biological Apocalypse.* Sandpoint, ID: Tetrahedron Pub. Group, 1999.

451 "Amazing Water." Interview with David Sereda. Amazing Water. Coast to Coast Am by George Noory. October 5, 2008.

452 Vachon, Marc, and Amy Vachon. *Equally Shared Parenting: Rewriting the Rules for a New Generation of Parents.* New York: Penguin Group, 2010.

453 Ken Keyes, *The Hundreth Monkey.* Coos Bay, Or.: Vision, 1987.

454 Abram Hoffer, Morton Walker, and Abram Hoffer. *Putting It All Together: The New Orthomolecular Nutrition.* New Canaan, CT: Keats, 1996.

455 Lepore, D. *The Ultimate Healing System*

456 Beddoe, A. F., and Jeanne Knight. Beddoe. *Biologic Ionization Applied to Farming and Soil Management: Principles and Techniques.* Oroville, WA: S & J Unlimited, 1997.

457 Beddoe and Knight, *Biologic Ionization*

458 Beddoe and Knight, *Biologic Ionization*

459 Preetha, P. P., V. G. Devi, and T. Rajamohan. "Hypoglycemic and Antioxidant Potential of Coconut Water in Experimental Diabetes." *Food Funct.* 3, no. 7 (July 3, 2012): 753-7. doi:10.1039/c2fo30066d.

460 Campbellfalck, D. "The Intravenous Use of Coconut Water." *The American Journal of Emergency Medicine* 18, no. 1 (January 2000): 108-11. doi:10.1016/S0735-6757(00)90062-7.

461 Beddoe and Knight, *Biologic Ionization*

462 M. T. Morter, *Your Health, Your Choice: Your Complete Personal Guide to Wellness,* Nutrition & Disease Prevention. Hollywood, FL: Fell Publishers, 1990.

463 International Maize and Wheat Improvement Center. "CIMMYT & Dr. Norman Borlaug." CIMMYT & Dr. Norman Borlaug. 2013. Accessed October 12, 2013. http://www.cimmyt.org/en/who-we-are?id=443:cimmyt-a-dr-norman-borlaug.

464 "The Many Headed Hydra of Gluten Sensitivity." Gluten Free Society. Accessed October 01, 2013. http://www.glutenfreesociety.org/gluten-free-society-blog/the-many-heads-of-gluten-sensitivity/.

465 Vojdani, A., T. O'Bryan, J.A. Green, J. McCandless, et al. "Immune Response to Dietary Proteins, Gliadin and Cerebellar Peptides in Children with Autism." *Nutritional Neuroscience* 7, no. 3 (June 1, 2004): 151-61. doi:10.1080/10284150400004155.

466 Mackenzie, D.L. "Variation in populations of enteral microflora in people with coeliac disease following the implementation of a gluten free diet: a thesis in partial fulfillment of the requirements for the degree of Master of Science in Human Nutrtion through the Institute of Food, Nutrtiions, and Human Health at Massey University, Palmerston, North New Zealand. 2008. URI. http://hdl.handle.net/1017903).

467 Mark Sircus, A.C. *Principles and Practices of Natural Allopathic Medicine.* Epub. Accessed October 10, 2013. http://drsircus.com/books/e-book/natural-allopathic-medicine/.

468 Clark, Hulda Regehr. *The Cure for All Cancers: With 100 Case Histories.* San Diego, CA: ProMotion Pub., 1993.

469 "The Many Headed Hydra of Gluten Sensitivity." Gluten Free Society. Accessed October 01, 2013. http://www.glutenfreesociety.org/ gluten-free-society-blog/the-many-heads-of-gluten-sensitivity/.

470 *PDR for essential oils* [S.I.]: Essential Science Pub., 1999.